The Curly Hair Book: Or How Men Can Now

MW00900324

Copyright © 2013 Ro

Table of Contents

Preface

This book that you are reading is the result of my many years experimenting, testing, trialling and researching all about hair, with a personal focus on curly hair as this is the hair texture that I have.

When I decided to write this book, I made it my objective to provide a literary resource that would bring an overall solution: to enable a male with curly hair to be satisfied with his hair. As it is, the vast majority of men with waves, coils and kinks remain in an oblivious stupor when it comes to their curly hair, regarding their genetically-determined shapely hair as a curse and a liability.

I too used to lack the knowledge and attitude to make something positive of my hair, and I would prefer to forget about my hair with a neat and self-imposed buzz cut instead of facing my then-perceived weakness. As a teenager who would prefer to conform to the silliness of regarding one's curly hair as a personal trait best forgotten about, I spent much of my life's early years in said stupor and not addressing that which would, years later, become a much-valued asset of mine and part of who I was.

Some 11 years ago, I decided that I had enough, and the teenager who had a bushy beast for hair embarked on a journey to successfully decipher and manage the stuff growing atop his head. Over a decade later, I find myself at peace with my curly hair and enjoying the life benefits obtained from having transformed a perceived weakness into a valuable strength. Something as trivial as making the most of one's hair can bring so much benefit because, after all, hair is a trait that is instantly recognised by others, hence the absurdity of not making the most of such follicular belonging.

I am satisfied with my curly hair, and now I want to bring the possibility for others to achieve this same satisfaction. Thus, this book encompasses all to do with curly hair for men and provides a solution that has been long needed. Specifically to you, this book will open a new door and enable you to finally be satisfied and proud of your curly hair as you will get to not only know it and manage it but to also regard your curly hair as a trait of yours with much potential.

This book has been a long-term project of mine, and a lot has happened during the timespan that this book has taken to be written and published. I have written this book in 4 countries, in different scenarios, with different moods, at different times of the day and so much more, so this book certainly carries many memories. Needless to say, writing this book has been a great experience that I have thoroughly enjoyed, and it is an honour to now be able to share this book with you. If there's one thing that I can assure you at this stage, it is that you will not regret reading this book.

Let's proceed.

Acknowledgements

In my life, I have always strived to surround myself with the best people, and this book would not have been possible if it wasn't for certain individuals. Ergo, before continuing with my book, I would like to publicly thank all of you who have given me your love, kindness and friendship during all our years together. Furthermore, I would like to specifically thank the following people:

- <u>You:</u> first of all, I'd like to thank you. Thank you for buying this book. With this purchase, you are placing your trust in me; you are coming to me for answers, and I have ensured to deliver those answers. I've written this book for you: this book is the guide, the manual and the blueprint for the modern male who simply wants to finally get his curly hair in order; it's a book for guys like you and I. Starting from the core concept of delivering results with convenience, I have written the following +230 pages for you, and I'm 100% confident that you will enjoy this book while learning and putting your acquired knowledge to good use. Thank you.

- <u>My parents:</u> it doesn't matter that for the last 11 years, I have been thousands of miles away from you guys; I've never felt that the distance that separated us was an impediment to feeling the love that only a father and a mother can give. Not even if I filled this book with millions of "thank yous", would that be enough to express my gratitude for what you have done for me. Regardless; mother, father: thank you.

I would also like to give a big shoutout to Tabrez, the man behind the cool cover for this book. You blew my mind when you sent me the first draft of the book cover after I had sent you my awfully-drawn sketch with the idea that I had in mind. A talented graphic designer, Tabrez is the owner of <u>This Is Cloud</u>, a high-quality graphic/website designing company, and I highly recommend his services. You can contact him directly at

tabrez@thisiscloudstudio.com

Finally, this book is dedicated to my dearly-missed grandmother, Josefa "Omapepi" (1927-1999), one of the strongest persons that I have ever had the pleasure to know. Rest in peace, Oma.

The Beginning Of A Revolution

"Just keep it short and tamed", said the barber.

I had asked him what haircut he recommended outside of the usual buzzing of my curls.

"Curly hair like yours is best kept tamed; it's a big hassle to keep it looking good. So, you want a #2 or are you going with a #3 this time?" he asked as he prepared both guards while the hair clipper stood motionless on the cabinet in front of me.

I was sitting in the barber chair and looking at my half-inch curls in the mirror; they were to be gone in a few minutes. Paradoxically, I was tired of buzzing my curls all the time, yet I kept coming back for more. Same haircut, same hairstyle, same everything.

"All right, let's go with the usual, a #2 all around", I replied, mumbling my words with a pessimistic voice as if I had lost some form of follicular battle.

Fast-forward to exactly 3 days later. It's Thursday evening, and I am sitting on the sofa browsing channels on TV, bored out of my mind as the weather is bad outside and I don't have anything better to do. It's 2001, so we didn't have Facebook or Twitter back in those days to entertain our spare time with.

I browse the channels without finding anything worth wasting my time on. I am about to call it quits when I notice a guy with blonde curls bouncing around on some silly talent show. I pause on this channel, intrigued by what my eyes are seeing. It is one of those talent TV shows in which people are chosen according to how good they can sing; hardly the stuff that I would otherwise consider dedicating even 10 seconds of my spare time to.

The blonde dude who caught my eyes is being interviewed after he had been selected to enrol the show. I don't pay attention to what he is saying as he is being interviewed, nor do I care for that matter; I am just weirdly fascinated by his curly hair. His curls are about 2 inches in length, dark blonde, perfectly moulded to fit his head; his curly hair in awesome synergy with his style and image. I could not stop gazing at the TV screen.

One of my brothers comes along, sits on the other sofa and asks me to change the channel.

"Why are you watching a cheesy show about people who claim to be singers?" he asked.

"I just had a revelation", I replied, this time with the brightest of eyes and as if I had discovered the truth to a deeply-hidden secret.

Fast-forward again, now to about 11 years after I had this revealing episode. I am writing a book, and it is not a book I would have thought 11 years ago that I would have decided to write. But then, this 11-year gap hasn't been what I'd considered a normal gap: I have been fortunate enough to so far have lived in 5 countries while developing my career, travelling around the world, meeting plenty of people, discovering new cultures and, of course, experimenting, trialling and testing everything on my curly hair and the waves, coils and kinks of other men.

After 11 years, I can say that I am happy with my curly hair and that I know all I need to know to have it looking as I desire. As a modern guy living in a fast-paced society, I want results, and I want those results to come with convenience. I certainly don't like wasting my time, and I like to look good too. My curly hair is part of my image, and it needs to look good without costing me my testosterone levels or inciting me to watch repeat episodes of <u>Sex in the City</u>. I like to wake up, have a quick shower, groom my curls and be out the bathroom in less than 10 minutes, ready to put on some clothes, grab my stuff for the day and leave my house satisfied with the stuff atop my head. And that's precisely what this book is all about.

All of my hair-related experience and lessons learnt are in this book. Everything good that has come out of my years of hacking my way into the pursuit of mastering curly hair is here. This book will show you how to groom and care after your waves, coils or kinks, and, just as importantly, it will instil in you the right attitude to have when it comes to sporting great curly hair without having to become a hair diva or spend your free time in hair salons surrounded by women gossiping about hot guys.

Having a great-looking head of curls as a male is not as difficult as you may have been made to believe, and the ultimate goal of this book is to offer you the until-now-unknown option of incorporating great curly hair into your life without having to sacrifice your lifestyle as a 21st century male. I have made it my personal goal to make this book your blueprint to great curly hair and show you everything to make your waves, coils or kinks a precious asset that will forever enhance your looks, confidence and overall life.

Are you ready?

1) Introduction: The Start Of An Awesome Mane Journey

"A man who dares to waste one hour of time has not discovered the value of life"

Charles Darwin

Why this book?

Because I have been in your place.

For many years, I went about my life without knowing what to do with my curly hair. Some days, I'd be able to tame it and put it into submission; other days my curly hair would just do whatever it wanted to do. I was never able to grow my curly hair more than a mere inch in length because doing so implied too much effort and dramas when it came to managing my mane. At the end of the day, I'd choose to sport my curly hair in a buzz cut and forget about it.

The thing is, curly hair is awesome. It really is. Curly hair comes in all shapes and forms: from smooth waves to unimaginable coils to exotic kinks. In reality, curly hair is just the umbrella term for all the types of hair that do not grow straight hence the multiple expressions available with curly hair. Regardless of the type, curly hair will enhance the image of its fortunate owner when looked after properly, yet most wavy, coiled and kinky haired men remain clueless as to how to groom and wear their manes optimally. We curly men lack optimal information on curly hair specific to our male needs, and we also lack inspiration from both popular curly men and average curly Joes who would otherwise motivate the rest of us to do something about our own locks. No wonder the vast majority of curly haired fellas are clueless about their hair!

While it is true that some popular curly haired dudes like Adrian Grenier, Justin Timberlake or Lenny Kravitz have all great curls, they also have enough money to be able to hire their own expert team of stylists and image consultants to do the hair care job for them. Many times, however, these popular men become dependent on image professionals to get their manes looking the part, and depending on other people is never the best way to go about in life. I always say that, if you want things done properly, it is you who must do them, not others.

Being able to make the most of our curly hair as males living modern lives becomes quite the trick: we lack optimal information on our hair texture, and the dudes whom we look up to for inspiration and as social reference are not always the best examples since the reality tends to be distorted in many of their cases. All of this is why I made it my goal to write a book in which I specifically and extensively covered everything to do with curly hair for men; a book written by a curly dude for curly dudes.

With The Curly Hair Book: Or How Men Can Now Rock Their Waves, Coils And Kinks, you will learn how to manage and groom your curly hair, and you will get your mane rocking all by yourself with the convenience and attitude that we 21st century males need as we live in this modern, hectic world. The end result of all this is what I have termed the "awesome mane" concept.

An awesome mane is more than just great-looking curly hair. An awesome mane is the result of knowing how to manage your curly hair and integrating it into your image, personality and life, which ultimately allows you to be truly satisfied with your hair. When you have an awesome mane, you have discarded any conventional notions of taming your hair with a buzz cut and you have fought the hair ignorance that unfortunately populates most curly males' minds. Because an awesome mane is based on knowledge, its achievement will allow you to reap the many benefits of having great-looking curls as you add another positive element to your life, and, since a good life is all about achieving success after success, you will be able to work towards an even better life with your newly-achieved success: your awesome mane. Sounds too elaborate and complex? Well, it's as simple as putting the knowledge you acquire in this book into actions, and you will soon have your awesome mane on autopilot.

This book will show you the tidbits of curly hair; it will teach you how to groom, manage and look after your curls, and it will enable you to live your life with an awesome mane. What's more is that I have written this book with YOU in the back of my mind at all times: this book is not a hair diva book, this book is not written by someone who doesn't know anything about living life as a modern male, and this book will not bore you to death with what you'd otherwise regard as girly content. I am a male, I have curly hair, and I have a goal: to help you achieve your awesome mane.

Who am I?

First and foremost, I am a dude with curls, just like you. Specifically, I have thick coils and kinks growing on my head: the top of my head and most of the sides and back have tight coils growing, while my nape and lower sides have much tighter coils (i.e. kinks). Essentially, I have Type III and IV curls, but don't worry about these numbers for now as you will learn all about the nomenclature of curly hair in the next chapter.

Some 11 years ago, I decided to cut through the nonsense and lack of optimal knowledge that surrounded curly hair for us men, and I embarked on an experimental journey to finally master the stuff that flourished from my scalp. I am the kind of guy who has always emphasised grabbing life by the horns and riding it; my curly hair was one of those elements in my life that was running wild and rampant 11 years ago, and it was then that I decided that it was time to address those rebellious locks. Through my peculiar awesome mane journey, I have learnt to manage and integrate my curly locks into my urban, active and 21st century modern lifestyle; a feat that would not have been possible had I not embarked on my hair-hacking journey over a decade ago.

In these 11 years, I've managed to live in 5 countries and travel to many more as having an international lifestyle is a choice that I made at the same time that I decided to embark on this awesome mane journey. In fact, my decision to go on to hack my hair conundrum was part of a series of decisions that I made when I was still a teenager and that had very deep existential connotations. Thus, I not only embarked on a hair-hacking journey but also on a life-enriching journey as I packed my bags, kissed my parents goodbye and went on to experience life as an adventure that would mature me into an overall better man. The only thing I knew for sure back then was that, during my whole adventure, my scalp would continue to grow naturally-curving hair strands no matter what.

During all these years, I've had my fair amount of battles with my hair; an ordeal that was a prerequisite to learning all about curly hair and that was at its everest before I started my hair-hacking journey. I was the one with voluminous curly hair that would grow like a bush as soon as it hit 1 inch in length, hence much of my early life was spent seeing my hair as a liability. As you read at the beginning of this book, it wasn't until I became inspired by another dude with an awesome mane that I decided, there and then, to do something about my hair; if he could do it, I surely could do it too.

The above was 11 years ago, and since then I have experimented with my hair in all forms and manners while studying it and helping others improve their curls too. In the name of experimentation and knowledge seeking, I have put the smelliest of gooey concoctions on my hair, I have grown my mane to reach my nipples and beyond, I have gone long periods of time without using any hair products on my curls, and I have blended all sort of ingredients to make potions to apply to my hair and the hair of others. The results have ranged from awesome to potentially dangerous, and I have acquired invaluable knowledge on curly hair through my peculiar journey.

With all the knowledge that I acquired over the years, I was able to finally get my curly hair to look as I wanted it to look, and, equally important, I learnt to embrace that which was inherent to me. There was no more lying to myself by rejecting what was unique to me with all those frequent visits to the barber to crop my hair because I didn't know what to do with my curvy locks. Instead, my acquiring of hair-specific knowledge allowed me to leave my house in the morning with my curly hair looking exactly as I wanted it to, and, of course, this achievement had a positive impact on my looks, self-confidence and overall quality of life. What was even better was that I was able to sport my awesome mane without having to spend countless hours in the bathroom or hair salon.

As I continued my journey, I was able to perfect the approach to achieving an awesome mane so that it would relate to my lifestyle as a male: I go to the gym, I like to be groomed and dressed in 20 minutes sharp, I like to go out with my friends to watch football, and I like to team up with my pals to play rugby. As a modern male, results must come with convenience, which is precisely what I know that you too value.

Despite all my hair-related experience, I am neither a hairdresser nor a barber, and I don't pretend to be one. Of course, I have done my fair amount of consulting with a good number of these hair professionals over the years, but cutting hair is an art best left to those who have plenty of hands-on experience trimming and shaping manes. Unfortunately for us curly dudes, many of these same professionals are taught from a straight-hair perspective, which consequently yields an overall lack of specific knowledge of curly hair by those whom we curly haired consumers reach out to for hair advice. In fact, one of the issues I had in the beginning of my hair-hacking journey was actually finding hair professionals who were knowledgeable in the field of curly hair for men.

In addition to the above, I tried reading as much as I could online and offline about hair as it related to us males with wavy, coiled and kinky hair, yet all I could find was advice that was either for women, emasculating, approached from a straight-hair perspective (and thus faulty) or was the same copy-and-paste rubbish that those annoying spamming websites like to regurgitate. All of this was back in the first years of our previous decade, and this misfortune still continues to this day except for a peculiar website that has preceded this book that you are reading.

Enter Manly Curls.

Chances are that you have read or heard about me before buying this book. This is because, for some time now, I have been leading and paving the online path for curly men to finally do something about their waves, coils and kinks. Before I started my website (Manly Curls), I had already been helping out guys offline with their curls for some years, but it was in May 2011 that I decided to make it my goal to reach men globally through the use of the Internet. Amidst a sea of useless hair-related content for curly haired men, I started Manly Curls, and, soon enough, I was reaching men from all backgrounds and nations. Then, the emails saying thank you started pouring in, and I knew factually that I had entered my desired journey of spreading the word worldwide and helping fellow curly haired men with their waves, coils and kinks on a global scale. This book is the next step in my current journey.

With this book, I want to bring you the wisdom and knowledge that I have acquired through the years on everything to do with curly hair so that you too can achieve your awesome mane. By finally embracing and doing something positive about your curly hair, you will be able to reap the many benefits that come from not only getting your curls to look like you want them to look but that also come from striving to better yourself as a male. Through my personal experience and my experience helping others, I can guarantee you that achieving an awesome mane, as you will be learning in this book, will ultimately have an immense carryover to your life, which as modern men is the kind of stuff that we welcome in our lives.

The curly hair paradigm

I call my curly hair my "beast". It is a nickname that I gave it when I first started experimenting with my hair. I was at university and dating a girl who was studying psychology, and she told me that naming the source of my dramas would help me embrace and address my then-perceived weakness, so I chose a name that totally represented what my curls liked to do on a daily basis. Through the years, the nickname has stuck although I would say that nowadays my beast is more akin to a cool and loyal Labrador dog keen to bring me the newspaper on a Sunday morning; that's how obedient my curly hair has become.

From a practical point of view and in terms of hair textures, humans have either straight hair or curly hair growing from their scalp. Curly hair is merely hair that grows in a non-straight pattern (i.e. it curls), and curly hair can curl slightly as it grows (i.e. wavy hair), curl in very tight coils or kinks (i.e. kinky hair) or anything in between! Thus, curly hair is the umbrella term covering the range of hair-curling expressions available, and it can be classified in 5 types as you will learn later on.

The reasons behind curly hair being expressed in so many curling patterns are not fully known; what is known is that a person's unique genetic makeup is to "blame" for having curly hair. Some explanations have been proposed as to how and why curly hair forms its characteristic curling pattern as it grows from the hair follicles, but the precise reasons have yet to be unveiled. I am pretty sure that scientists have more important things to do than decipher the intricacies of curly hair, so the take-home message is that curly hair grows in a non-straight pattern right from its very inception (i.e. the follicle), which then allows for the many types that curly hair can express itself in. So yeah, we've got curly hair, and it's about time that we do something positive about it.

Before we continue, let me say that straight hair is as great as curly hair. Hair is just hair, and you'd be a fool to view yourself as better or worse than someone with the opposite hair texture. However, the approach to managing curly hair is different and more elaborate than that of straight hair, and the advice available to us curly haired men when it comes to hair grooming is biased from a straight-hair perspective because straight hair is easier to style and manage.

You see, because of the inherent bending shape and curving pattern of our waves, coils and kinks, we curly men are predisposed to having dry and tangled hair. Our curls also tend to defy gravity no matter how long we grow them, and trying to use a hairbrush or regular comb to style our manes is a recipe for disaster. We also don't respond as well as straight hair to conventional hair products, and the look we sport when our curly hair is damp differs wildly from the look that our mane has once it has fully dried. Not only does curly hair require a more careful grooming approach than straight hair does but curly hair can also be quite an inconvenience to have if one doesn't know how to manage it properly.

All of the above is what leads the majority of curly men to give up on their hair and regard it as a curse of some sorts; I know this very well because I was like that too. We curly men have viewed our hair as something unexplainable and as something that cannot be understood. We are constantly bombarded with images of men with awesome straight haired manes, yet we cannot relate to them because our hair is just not like that. We read men's magazines with hair advice and cool hairstyle options that don't work for us in real life because the advice is written from a straight-hair perspective and assumption. Thus, we prefer to tame our beasts with frequent visits to the barber to get ourselves a buzz cut and forget about an inherent trait of ours that comes naturally.

This curly hair paradigm is not only specific to men; curly women have also had an enduring battle with all this straight hair baloney. The equivalent of our buzz cuts to women is the straightening of their curls. From relaxers to hair-straightening gadgets, women are brainwashed to tame their curls and keep them straight. Straight hair is docile, and being docile is, after all, how we are expected to behave in our modern-day societies.

Overall, curly hair remains somewhat of a mystery to us curly men. We own it, but we don't know it. We live with it every day, but we reject it and prefer to forget about its existence. Of course, if we go through life with such a view on our hair, it is then only normal that the vast majority of curly haired men won't be knowing anything about the stuff that populates their heads. And, when it comes to your curly hair, you should skip mysteries and instead strive to know all about your curls because, by doing so, you will be able to make the most of that which is innately yours and which should never be deemed as negative.

The Awesome Mane concept

An awesome mane is not just about having great-looking curly hair. An awesome mane is curly hair that has been taken beyond mediocrity and that symbolises a positive attitude to oneself and to one's overall life. The Awesome Mane concept digs into the core of a male's need to better himself in order to maximise his potential. It rehashes the perspective of curly hair from that of a seemingly trivial and negative trait to that of a valuable asset that is an integral piece of the puzzle that makes you as a male, with this puzzle being, what I call, the self-puzzle.

An awesome mane carries an attitude that defies conventional notions and that is strong and solid in its foundation. An awesome mane implies embracing what you have, not looking for excuses, and making the most of that which you were born with. An awesome mane is just one more piece of the overall puzzle that constructs your identity (i.e. your self-puzzle).

At its core, an awesome mane has a physical part and a mental part that need to be addressed concomitantly:

1) Physical part: the hair-specific aspects relating to grooming and caring that will yield the cosmetic benefits and the great-looking hair.

2) Mental part: the attitude and lifestyle aspects relating to taking positive action with regards to one's hair and using the achievement of great hair as a way to maximise one's potential as a male.

Figure 1 – The 2 parts to an awesome mane

AWESOME MANE	
Physical	*Mental*
Hair grooming	Attitude
Hair care	Social references
Haircut/Hairstyle	Inspiration
Hair accessories	Motivation
Hair products	Self-puzzle enhancement

All of this is what distinguishes an awesome mane, as trivial as it may be, as a symbol of success and achievement. Sure, having an awesome mane entails having a great-looking mane of curls atop your head, but there is also an attitude and an approach required to having a great-looking curly mane as a modern male living in a society that wants gullible and opiated sheep, yet is in dire need of men who can think for themselves. Thus, in this book, you will not only find the part pertaining to all there is to achieving a great set of curls but you will also find the part that develops and ingrains the positive and strong mentality needed to achieve and own an awesome mane.

From the first day that I decided to get myself an awesome mane, I knew that I needed a change in attitude to my hair and even life. We, modern males, have lost our need to be leaders and thinkers, character traits that were once essential to thrive in this world. Our modern jobs require us to be docile and to adhere to what we are ordered to do. At home, we have a TV brainwashing us to imitate other people and buy stuff that we don't need. We go online and have, at the click of a button, a whole second world in which to lose ourselves, all while we happily conform to a life of monotony and obedience. Instead of coming up with our own principles, we take the principles and life attitudes thrown at us by trendy films, flashy magazines and even bar talk. Due to our exposure in today's society to so many conforming messages and submissive lures, we carry the same passive attitude to everything in our lives, including our curly hair.

To achieve your awesome mane, you have to be a man. A man of principles, beliefs and determination. A man who embraces what he has and who always goes with what he deems best after having evaluated it thoroughly. In essence, you must address your awesome mane as part of the territory of being a man and not a pseudo male as society wants us to be.

An awesome mane will instantly improve your looks and image, which in turn will give you more self-confidence, and the self-confidence achieved will ultimately better your life. In fact, by starting with your awesome mane and realising the benefit of making the most of what you have, you will be able to apply the same self-embracing concept and attitude of an awesome mane to the rest of your life. By addressing and improving the smallest pieces of your self-puzzle, such as your hair, you will be able to see how you can use the improving of these trivial pieces as potential tools to maximise your self-confidence and self-belief. This constant self-actualising emphasis will allow you to enjoy the confidence carryover that constantly improving yourself will have on your life.

When you get to experience for yourself the immense carryover obtained by achieving your awesome mane, you will be able to become inspired and motivated to work on improving the rest of your physique, your social skills, your personal relations, your health and the other facets and elements of your personal existence, which once bettered will lead to a progressive enhancement of your self-puzzle and life. I want you to regard the pursuit of your awesome mane as a life-enriching goal that, once achieved, will help you to become an overall better man.

An awesome mane is not determined by a specific hair length or curl type. Any men can have an awesome mane: a guy with wavy hair, kinky hair, long hair, short hair or even a balding head. The concept of an awesome mane is all about making the most of your curls regardless of length, type, form or quantity. You embrace what is unique to you, and you do something positive about it. Simple.

Thus, the goal for you is to embark on a journey to achieve your awesome mane, and you will have concluded this journey when you are finally happy with your hair. There are no objective markers or sets of measures that define the achievement of your awesome mane; this is not a competition, nor is this a business plan to show to a company's board of directors. This is a goal you set yourself to achieve because you want to make the most of your curly hair; once you are happy with how your hair looks and with how it has been customised to your self-puzzle, you will have then accomplished your awesome mane. Nothing more, nothing less.

In the many pages that are to come, I bring you the knowledge, inspiration, motivation and attitude needed to achieve your own awesome mane; ultimately, however, it will be you who finishes the journey and achieves the goal of an awesome mane, going on to add yet another success to your life.

Why are awesome manes so uncommon?

Simply put, because of lack of information and inspiration. I will talk about this further in the book, but the reason behind the difficulty in finding curly men with awesome manes is that there is simply a lack of information and inspiration going around for us to retrieve.

Before I started my website, the curly dudes that came to me for advice all complained about the same:

"I wish there was more information on how to care after my hair."

"I'd try to do something about my curly hair if only the hair care information that I read didn't make me feel like I was part of the cast of Sex in the City."

"I wish I didn't have to go to an expensive hair salon full of ladies with tin foil on their hair to be able to sport a good set of curls."

"I wish there were more men going around with great-looking curly hair so that I could become inspired."

"Is curly hair really that bad? I hardly see any curly men with good hair."

What's more is that as soon as I started my website and because I could now reach with my words to a larger worldwide audience, I would get dozens and dozens of emails per week of men who would thank me for finally creating an online space for curly men to visit and get the knowledge they much needed to finally do something about their hair.

It is only normal though. If you don't have access to optimal information on curly hair, you just won't do anything about your particular waves, coils or kinks. Since the vast majority of men with the same limited access to information as yourself are not going to do anything positive about their curls, then there will hardly be any inspiration going around when it comes to an awesome mane. It's a vicious cycle, and it is one that I aim to break with this book.

To top the above, men are brainwashed to believe that it is only females who can have good hair. With us men, it seems as though hair mentality is still stuck in the early 20th century. Conventional notion says that men should tame their hair and anyone doing otherwise is labelled as "different" (that's if they are lucky). Well, guess what? Going against conventional notion is not wrong, provided that it is done with self-belief, confidence and assertiveness. If it weren't for those men who dared to be different, the aircraft industry would have never developed as rapidly as it did in the early 20th century as Orville and Wilbur Wright (aka the Wright brothers) would not have insisted in their pioneering desire to defy gravity. If it were because being different is bad or wrong, Sir Richard Branson would have never dared to rehash the music industry in the early '70s and proceed to build the massive business empire he currently owns; I guess that if he had preferred to not be different, he'd still continue to happily trade in the same small record shop that he started in and would have left it at that.

Fact is, being oneself, thinking for oneself and sticking to one's principles and beliefs is the way to go for a successful life and, of course, for an awesome mane.

The opposite of an awesome mane: dead rats and buzz cuts

Enter the "dead rat" concept.

The "dead rat" is the opposite of an awesome mane in terms of hair knowledge; you know the kind of hair that I am talking about. Like you, I have tried growing my locks over an inch in length, and I would always end up sporting what looked like a dead rat on top of my head. Thankfully, my dead rat would not last very long because I am lucky to have some stylish friends who would be able to tell me right away when my hair looked like a dead rat. Unfortunately, not all guys are lucky to have these same stylish friends or are as receptive to hair criticism as myself, hence one gets to see dead rats much more often than awesome manes when it comes to male curly hair. Thus, a dead rat is awful-looking hair that has been caused by its owner's lack of specific hair knowledge.

Then, you have the "buzz cut" concept.

The "buzz cut" is the opposite of an awesome mane in terms of attitude. The buzz cut is the haircut of those curly haired men who force themselves to hit the barber every X amount of weeks to get a neat buzz cut or very short cut because they want to forget about their manes as they regard their hair in a negative manner. They don't ignore and tame their manes because they inherently like a buzz cut (although some do); no, they get a buzz cut because they plainly dislike their hair as they don't know what to do with it (remember my introductory story at the barber?). By all means, a buzz cut looks great in some men (especially for kinky haired men), but a buzz cut should be just another haircut/style option of the many possible for an awesome mane. I like to jokingly relate getting a buzz cut to self-castrating oneself because imposed buzz cuts represent the contrary of the manliness and self-confidence that an awesome mane exudes.

The world is full of dead rats and buzz cuts. Lack of information and lack of inspiration are behind all this curly hair negativity, so set the attitude to your hair straight (no pun intended), and fight those tempting dead rats and buzz cuts with an awesome mane!

An awesome mane is for men of all ages and background

Any men can have his awesome mane, it doesn't matter where you come from or who you are. I have met plenty of men with awesome manes from diverse backgrounds, and, coincidentally yet expectedly, the traits that they all shared were that they were men of mental fortitude and were worthy of admiration.

Through my international travels, I have found that neither culture nor nationality are impediments to an awesome mane; nor is age nor is religion nor is race, for that matter. This book is intended for people like you and I, though I cannot know for certain who reads my words. I don't know you, but one thing I do know is that you and I share the same interest in having an awesome mane, and I can tell you right now, in this precise moment, that you too can achieve and have your awesome mane and add another success to your life.

Lastly, having an awesome mane is independent of age. Sure, someone in his teens will differ in taste as to how he wants his awesome mane to look when compared to a curly fellow in his 50s. An awesome mane is not about hairstyles or about following trends; an awesome mane is about acknowledging and making the most of your curls, and that, my friend, has no boundaries.

The 5 rules of an awesome mane

The following 5 rules are the pillars to an awesome mane, and it is in your interest to abide by them at all times as they will make the journey easy and fast and will preserve your awesome mane for the rest of your life:

1) <u>You will have the right attitude</u>

It all starts with you. You can't change your genes or how your scalp decides to grow the shape of your hair. You've got curly hair; accept it and face it. Instead of defeating yourself with a pessimistic attitude, look at it from the bright side: you are capable of growing stuff that has the potential to change your image, make you unique, skyrocket your looks and inspire others.

The right attitude implies positivity, determination and assertiveness; hardly the qualities that sell millions on TV or in magazines. Bear these qualities in mind at all times when reading this book because you don't just need the knowledge to have great-looking curly hair; you also need the attitude. Otherwise, stop reading right now and don't waste your time with the next dozens and dozens of pages of awesome mane knowledge. Go to the barber, get your usual buzz cut and get on with your usual life.

2) <u>You will drop all conventional notions and stereotypes</u>

To achieve your awesome mane, you will only need this book, nothing more. You won't have to browse endless websites or magazines to try and decipher the code to making something positive of your curly hair. Discard everything you thought you knew about curly hair, and start fresh and with a reset brain to be able to absorb what is to come and learn how to finally achieve a great-looking head of curls the right way.

Following from the above, drop all stereotypes: looking after your hair is neither girly nor feminine. I have made it my personal goal to never put your testosterone levels at risk in the name of good hair, and you will not have to befriend your hairdresser so that he/she quotes you a better price to give you fabulous hair. In fact, you will be reading later on about a routine that has you in and out of the bathroom in just under 9 minutes. That's 9 minutes from the moment that you get in the shower to the moment that you are out of the bathroom with your awesome mane all set and ready to take the day. That's hardly girly, don't you think?

3) You will use and apply the optimal knowledge and tool

If it were as simple as me telling you to get in the shower, shampoo your curls, jump out of the shower and comb your hair, then I would not have needed to write a whole book on the topic of curly hair. Fact is, it is a bit more complicated than that, but it can be perfectly done by a modern male living a busy life full of successes. This book is lengthy, and I extensively cover every aspect of achieving an awesome mane so as to give you all the knowledge you need. Once you acquire all the knowledge in this book, the management of your awesome mane will become second nature, and you will have finally made the most of such a personal piece of your self-puzzle. Thus, this book is your tool, and inside you will find the optimal knowledge.

4) You will inspire others

The inspiration going around for an awesome mane is scarce. When you are carrying your awesome mane proud, when you are walking around with your curly hair looking good, when you leave your house happy with what you have atop your head, you have accepted to enter a silent gentlemen's agreement: to inspire others who, as you once did, have problems of any measure with their curly hair. This doesn't mean that you have to become a help desk or that you have to start a website with Q&As, not at all.

This gentlemen's agreement consists of inspiring others in any form or manner with your awesome mane. This can be in the form of inspiring others by not even saying a word as you walk with your awesome mane and other curly men are able to see for themselves that having a great head of curls is quite possible and doable. It can also be in the form of another curly dude approaching you and asking you a question (this will happen sooner or later) and you trying to give him some pointers to help him out. It doesn't matter, what matters is that, by having an awesome mane, you will automatically be a source of inspiration to others as you will be noticed everywhere you go by fellow curly men.

5) You will be a better man

A real man does all possible to enhance his self-puzzle and live a better life. By achieving your awesome mane, you will be maximising something inherent to you without taking away from other areas of your life. Yes, you will finally get better hair, but never forget that you are doing this as part of becoming a better man. As you achieve your awesome mane, take advantage of the positive momentum created from seeing the desired positive changes in your hair, and continue to improve other areas of your life that are subpar. The same positive, determined and assertive attitude required to have an awesome mane is the one that is just as essential to improve the rest of your life.

Wrapping it all up

I deemed it necessary to introduce this book as I have in this chapter to prepare you for what is to come in the many pages of this book. The following chapter "Curly Hair 101: Know Your Waves, Coils Or Kinks" will have you immersing yourself with awesome mane stuff right from the very beginning, but I need you to first be 100% sure that you want to do this. Read this introductory chapter as many times as you need, take your time. Do not, however, skip to the next chapter until you are 100% sure that an awesome mane is what you want and that you are motivated to pursue it.

What you are about to read in the rest of this book will forever change your perspective towards your hair and will give you the knowledge to add another improvement and success to your life. You will be able to maximise something inherent to you and thus gain control of something that you had quite likely given up on before.

My words are aimed at achieving an awesome mane because I have been in exactly the same place as you are. I, like you, have the same appreciation for good hair and want an awesome mane that doesn't cost me my masculinity. I, like you, am a modern male with curly hair living in a society that wants submissive and passive men when what it really needs is people who can think for themselves. I, like you, have been confronted with stereotypes and lack of information and inspiration for my curly hair, yet, by abiding by my own principles and beliefs, I was able to do as I believed in and enhance my self-puzzle. All by simply working on something as trivial as hair.

The choice is now yours, my friend.

My personal experience

The Curly Hair Book: Or How Men Can Now Rock Their Waves, Coils And Kinks is based on my experience having, learning and living with curly hair while helping others maximise theirs too. This book is based on my experience mastering an asset that will be staying with me for too long to not be making the effort to know it fully. Some 11 years ago, I had a realisation: I wanted to do something about my curly hair and stop, once and for all, those dreaded buzz cuts. I was inspired in an instant by a dude on TV who had great curly hair, and it was then, in that moment, that I decided to embark on a hair-hacking journey.

I remember looking around for information so as to be able to fix the mess that I had for hair, but all I found was either hair advice aimed at women or hair advice written by straight haired dudes for straight haired dudes. It made sense though, straight hair is much easier to manage than curly hair, and we men don't like intricate hair grooming stuff anyway.

I remember enquiring my trusted barber about what I could do with my curly hair, and all he could recommend was to keep it short and neat (i.e. a buzz cut). Desperate for answers, I have also mistakenly accepted to sacrifice my testosterone levels by visiting hair salons packed with ladies drinking tea and eating biscuits while verbally drooling over the latest "hot guy" and where the hairdressers were keen to do all sort of complex stuff on my hair to make it look great. Of course, my mane would look great until I washed it the next morning, and then I would have to hit the hair salon again if I wanted the same great hair. This left me no other option than to experiment, and experiment (wildly) I did.

I am a thrill seeker by nature, so I was keen to experiment anyway. After all, and as I have written in this chapter already, if you want things done properly, it'd better be you the one who does them. I kept an open mind throughout this hair-hacking journey and rejected all conventional notions and stereotypes. I did feel a bit girly (for lack of a better word) applying blends of oils on my hair as I had to wait 30 minutes to see if they worked or not, but I would hit the gym extra hard that day to undo any girliness.

Every time I carried out an experiment, I would learn something new, and over the years I was able to acquire immense amounts of hair knowledge. Along the way, I have also helped many men improve their hair and achieve their awesome manes too. It got to a point that friends of friends would email me questions on what to do with their curly manes, and I decided to start my site, Manly Curls, so that I could share and spread the curly-hair word worldwide. As the popularity of my site increased, no longer were friends of friends the only ones contacting me for hair advice but also men from all over the world whom, of course, I would have never reached and known otherwise. All of this then prompted me to write the book that you are now reading.

All the awesome mane knowledge that I have accumulated throughout the years is here in this book. With this book, not only will you be gaining knowledge but you'll also be gaining time: you will be able to skip all the hair dramas and useless stuff that I went through to be able to acquire the knowledge that is needed for an awesome mane. I have focused my efforts on making this book your one and only reference for everything hair related, and I can assure you that making the decision to achieve your awesome mane will be the right step in your life, just like it was for me.

Before we move on to the next chapter, allow me to take a moment to quickly tell you how I have structured this book.

Every chapter follows from one another, and I recommend you to initially read the book without skipping chapters. The content that I have written is at times heavy in words, and I do reference content from previous chapters, hence the need for you to not skip chapters (at least for your first read) so that you can grasp every bit of advice and build on the knowledge flow. Some chapters will require you to read the content a few times, and that is all fine and dandy; I have gone in great length to write and document everything so that once you learn all the content in this book, you will be able to put your acquired knowledge on autopilot and have it become second nature. You will learn, for example, how to find your optimal shampooing frequency, so, really, there is a method to the madness!

I have also written this book with your reading convenience in the back of my mind at all times. You will have noticed by now that I do use actual numbers instead of spelling them (e.g. 2 instead of two) so that you can spot them easier. You've probably also noticed that I gravitate towards writing in British English (so I spell "-ise" instead of "-ize"); this only has to do with this variant being the most comfortable that I find myself in to write a book, though I have certainly aimed to keep a neutral tone of English throughout the book. Moreover, it is my goal for you to relate to my personal case because doing so will allow you connect with the knowledge better. Thus, you will find a style of writing that is friendly, close and casual, yet, at the same time, it is also catchy and straightforward.

Lastly, you will see that I start each chapter with an introduction, and then I follow with the in-depth explanations of the topic to be covered in the given chapter. I end each chapter by offering you my personal experience in the topic covered, telling you how it has related to me and how it has been of my benefit. I am the first one following what I preach, and, if I have written it in this book, it is because I have done it and found it to be of benefit and use to the awesome mane journey. Furthermore, I have included chapters that cover additional questions or miscellaneous content that you may find yourself asking as you initiate your awesome mane journey.

Overall, I have aimed to cover absolutely everything that there is to a great head of modern curls, and I regard The Curly Hair Book: Or How Men Can Now Rock Their Waves, Coils And Kinks as the tool that will engine a hopeful revolution of men sporting awesome manes and converting those with dead rats and buzz cuts!

Without further ado, I now bring you the next chapter: "Curly Hair 101: Know Your Waves, Coils Or Kinks".

2) Curly Hair 101: Know Your Waves, Coils Or Kinks

"An investment in knowledge pays a great dividend"

Benjamin Franklin

To achieve an awesome mane, you need to know that which flourishes on top of your head: your curly hair. This chapter deals with the physical part of an awesome mane, and it is your introduction to the 2 essential aspects of managing your curly hair: your hair grooming routine and your hair care strategy. These aforementioned 2 aspects will be specifically covered in great depth in the chapters devoted to them, so it is equally important for you to be introduced to your curly hair and know the basics of it.

There are 2 textures of hair, straight and curly, and a human will grow either straight hair or curly hair, albeit curly hair can be expressed in several types. Curly hair grows its expressed shape as genetically determined, so you are stuck with how it grows for the rest of your life. What's more is that, as a male, your hair has an expiration date, so it is imperative to act now and make the most of your hair while it lasts.

Your curly hair will be a specific curl type, and it will also be at a specific hair length. These 2 elements are the foundation of your curly hair knowledge, and both of them will become extremely relevant in your quest to achieving your awesome mane as you proceed to master your hair grooming and hair care. Thus, in this chapter, the priority is for you to know your curl type and your hair lengths (there's 2 of them) so as to be able to get the most of the following chapters and of your awesome mane efforts.

I must emphasise to you that acquiring an awesome mane need not be done like a hair diva, nor does it have to cost you your testosterone levels, so rest assured as you read this chapter that you can have a great-looking head of curls while continuing with your chosen lifestyle as a modern male. The trick lies in acquiring the attitude, knowledge and inspiration needed to achieve an awesome mane, so let's now proceed to dig deep into all there is about curly hair.

What is hair?

Hair is a type of biomaterial that our bodies produce to keep us warm and protect the skin. Hair that grows in the scalp is primarily composed of a protein called keratin, and the whole length of an individual hair is called a "strand". In the scalp, a single hair strand grows from a "follicle", a tiny pocket buried inside the scalp. The part of the hair strand that you see (i.e. the part protruding from the scalp) is commonly referred to as the "shaft", and it grows in a filamentous manner. Individual hair strands are most often found grouped together in "locks":

a typical hair strand in the scalp will grow in the same direction as the hair strands that are next to it, hence dozens of hair strands typically group together to grow in the same direction and make a single lock of hair.

The hair shaft is composed of 3 layers: the medulla (innermost layer), the cortex (layer covering the medulla) and the cuticle (outer layer covering the medulla). The cuticle is composed of overlapping dead cells laid like shingles on a roof, and the cuticle itself is the layer of the hair shaft that we feel when we touch a given hair strand and that protects and strengthens the shaft as a whole. From now on, do note that I will use in this book the terms "strand" and "shaft" in an interchangeable manner to refer to an individual hair piece, whereas I will use the term "lock" or "hair lock" to refer to a bunch of hair strands grouped together.

The process of how a hair strand grows is that new hair material is being continuously added to the hair shaft from inside the follicle. Thus, your hair effectively grows from the follicle, and any new hair growth will be visually manifested at the base of the hair shaft (i.e. the segment closest to the scalp); hair does not grow from the tips as some people think. The good thing about the manner in which hair grows is that your hair is growing at all times to produce fresh new segments in the hair strands, so, if you cut or damage your current hair, you know that you will eventually grow new segments of the same cut or damaged strands; otherwise, we'd still be stuck with any bleaching or embarrassing hair modifications that we did to our hair in our teens!

In terms of the basics of hair, there is another essential element that you must know of, and that is scalp "sebum". The same hair follicles that hair grows from also have tiny sacks attached to them (known as sebaceous glands) that continuously secrete a natural endogenous substance resembling an oil and which is known as sebum. This oily substance is designed to coat the hair shaft, and the purpose of the sebum is to strengthen the whole hair strand and protect it from the outside elements. The end result of optimal sebum coating of the hair strands is hair that is shiny and strong, looks full and vigorous, and exudes health. Ergo, having your hair coated in your own sebum (i.e. sebuminised) is key to having an awesome mane, but this doesn't happen on its own with curly hair, and the sebum needs to be spread manually (by you) to ensure its proper coating of the hair strands.

Figure 2 – Diagram of a follicle including a hair shaft, sebaceous glands and associated follicular tissue

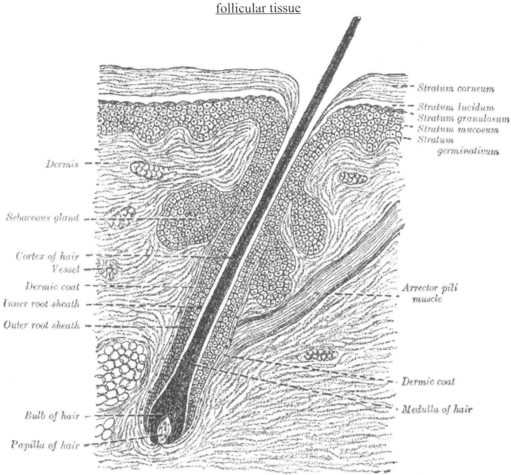

Hair has played an important role in our society since humans have inhabited the planet. The hair that grows from our scalp serves to protect our heads from the sun and environment, and it also serves to enhance our perceived attractiveness. Nowadays, since we have moved from caves to comfortable houses, the evolutionary role of hair has been practically lost as our exposure to the elements is much lower and beauty can be altered and faked in many ways. However, hair is still highly valued in our modern society for its beauty-enhancing properties in both women and men.

Men throughout history have worn their hair in different styles, manners and lengths, with hair coming to symbolise youth, physical vigour and prowess. From long hair to carefully-trimmed locks, men have used their hair as an indicator of their social and biological status since hair is a physical trait that is easily and instantly recognised. Centuries ago, and somewhat in present day too, if you wanted to look defiant or be feared, you'd grow your hair long, and, if you wanted to be taken as a man of class, you'd wear your hair short and neat.

Consequently, hair has played an important part in the social development of male status and role from past to present.

Male pattern baldness (MPB) is a type of balding almost exclusive to men, and it affects about 65% of men by age 60. MPB is a form of balding that is progressive, and it is categorised in 7 stages via the Hamilton-Norwood scale. The balding inflicted by MPB is irreversible and can hit a male at any age and of any background, although there is a strong genetic component associated to it. This is why it is so important that you do something about your hair now and learn how to achieve an awesome mane. I always say that, sooner or later, your hair will go, so it's in your interest to make the most of it while it lasts!

Lastly, hair grows, on average, 0.5 inches (or about 1 centimetre) per month, and the rate of hair growth is affected by your diet, hormonal status and overall health. While trying to speed up your hair growth process is quite an experimental endeavour, you can certainly and easily slow down your hair growth. Not having an optimal diet that promotes healthy hair growth, being seriously ill, or not having optimal levels of several bodily hormones can wreak havoc in the rate at which your hair grows as well as impair the quantity and quality of the hair strands.

Straight hair vs. Curly hair

Humans grow either straight hair or curly hair (i.e. non-straight hair) from the scalp. As you have learnt in the previous chapter, curly hair remains somewhat of a paradigm, nobody really knows for sure how and why it grows in a curled pattern: it is believed that the curving nature of curly-textured hair is caused by an uneven hair shaft structure as well as by a flat or oval cross-sectional shape of the hair shaft and follicle (it is round in straight hair), all of which is dictated by our genes. However, other than interesting explanations, what we know for sure is that the difference between straight hair and curly hair is that straight hair grows naturally and infinitely without curving at any length whereas curly hair curves and bends by default as it grows from the follicle. In other words, curly hair is non-straight hair, which gives rise to the different types of curly hair that we humans express, from smooth waves to springy coils to tight kinks and anything in between.

Many men don't know if they have straight or curly hair, let alone what type of curly hair they may have. This is why I like to make things as easy to understand as possible, and I have created a convenient curl typing guide based on how long it takes one's hair to form curls. This way, we can objectively categorise all the expressions of curly hair instead of using loose terms such as "wavy", "kinky", "rounded" or "coily", terms that cause unneeded confusion and detract us from finding optimal hair information.

Since the majority of men don't grow their hair beyond 2 inches in length, they also never get to know whether their hair truly curls or not as, for example, wavy hair can look straight at very short lengths, thus adding more confusion to the hair-learning effort. A good subjective hint, and one that I like to joke about, is that if you fear growing your hair beyond a mere 1 inch in length because it gets to look like a mushroom or because it is too annoying to look after, then chances are that you have curly hair. There's a pretty good reason for me lovingly calling my curly hair a beast!

Fortunately for our straight haired peeps, straight hair has it easy when it comes to looking its best. The aforementioned natural sebum secreted from the scalp travels all the way through the shaft of straight hair in a smooth and uninterrupted manner. Curly hair, on the other hand, curves and bends, which makes coating the hair strands with sebum more difficult to achieve across their entire length. Overall, the non-straight pattern of curly hair translates into this hair texture being more difficult to manage and the too-common scenario of having one's curls acting beastly if not looked after properly, with dead rats and buzz cuts becoming the norm once the beast mode strikes.

Indeed, it is said bending and curving of curly hair that has us, dudes with curls, having to endure our manes randomly gaining unwanted volume, looking totally different when they dry as opposed to when they were wet or damp, acting as if they had a life of their own and looking different every day. To top that, curly hair will curl at different lengths depending on its type, which means that the dramas that we experience with our curls will somewhat differ according to our specific type of curly hair too.

All of this was, some time ago, the reason for me deciding to sit down and come up with an easy-to-understand and useful typing guide for curly hair; a guide that will help you to identify your type of curly hair and that will serve you to define its management. While the vast majority of the curly hair advice in this book is generic and applicable to all curl types, there are also some tidbits that are specific to each type of curly hair and that will be covered together with said generic advice for curly hair.

The Curly Hair Type Guide

To reiterate what I wrote in the previous section, one can have either straight hair or curly hair growing from his scalp. Straight hair is hair that grows straight and doesn't show any curling/bending pattern as it grows. On the other hand, curly hair curves and bends, and, as it grows, it will form curls, albeit each male's curly mane will form its curls at unique and uniform vertical lengths. The ability for each male to grow curls at genetically-determined lengths specific to himself is the basis for our curl typing guide, the Curly Hair Type Guide, and its classification.

Essentially, curly hair can be classified in a spectrum of 5 types according to the vertical length at which a full curl is formed, with these types being expressed in Roman numbers: I, II, III, IV and V. Note that from here onwards, I will use "type of curly hair", "curly hair type" and "curl type" interchangeably to refer to any of the 5 types making up the spectrum of curly hair. Furthermore, the curl type classification ranges in the vertical length that it takes each curl type to form a full curl, and this range is a descending one in that Type I curly hair takes the longest vertical length to form a curl and Type V curly hair takes the shortest vertical length to form a curl. The term "tight" and "tightness" will be used to represent this decreasing vertical length the higher the curl type is, thus "tighter" curly hair will be the higher-end curl types (Type III, IV and V) whereas "looser" curly hair will be the lower-end curl types (Type I and II). Don't worry about it if this doesn't make sense at the moment; as you continue reading, it will fall into place neatly.

Curly hair can vary wildly in expressions, from what is colloquially known as wavy hair to tight pencil-thin coils to zig-zag kinks. A male always has a predominant curl type growing from his scalp although it is not uncommon to have 2 curl types concomitantly expressing on one's head (though there is always a predominant one). The difficulty lies in grouping similar expressions of curls into types so that we men can further define our awesome mane efforts according to our specific curly hair type. The vertical length at which a full curl is formed is an optimal grouping factor since a male's hair follicles produce curls at fairly uniform lengths as dictated by one's genetic makeup.

Through the popularity of my site, my curl typing guide is already used by plenty of men worldwide as a tool to approach the management of their curls, and it is a guide that I had already tested on other curly dudes' manes prior to publishing it online. This same curl typing guide will be extremely useful to you as you will be able to relate to your specific curl type while understanding its inherent needs. In fact, working out your curl type is of utmost value in achieving your awesome mane as not only does it allow you to actually classify your hair but it also allows you to approach your curls and awesome mane efforts without getting too girly or causing inconvenience on your part. All you need is a ruler and 5 minutes of your time, no testosterone or manhood will be sacrificed in the process.

The essence of the Curly Hair Type Guide is to put your curly hair into an established curl type so that you can have a starting point to your awesome mane path. This is because just going about throwing whatever products to your mane or styling your curls with whatever your lady has in the bathroom won't cut it if you want a great head of curls. On the latter, you can also use this curl typing guide with your (if you have) lady or partner and even your children so that you can all start sharing the same hair grooming and hair care approaches as well as any purchased hair products. An awesome mane doesn't know of ages and, dare I say, gender!

While knowing your curl type is of great use, the most important thing is that you are aware that your curly hair requires a different grooming and maintenance approach from that of straight hair, which is why you need specific knowledge outside that of the regurgitated straight hair content that we curly men are bombarded with online and offline. I have tailored this book around the premise of knowing your curly hair and taking appropriate actions, and your curl type is one of those elements that you must know so as to lay the groundwork for your awesome mane.

Factors to consider before identifying your curl type

Before learning how to measure your curls and how to identify your curl type, you must first be aware of several factors regarding this curl typing guide as it is quite likely that you are new to typing and profiling your hair.

Identifying your curl type is a very useful approach in that you will be able to put your hair into a specific group that shares peculiar awesome mane requirements. The vast majority of the content that you will encounter in this book is applicable to all curl types indistinctively, and the 2 main areas in which the advice for curly hair will differ slightly according to your curl type is in the defining of your hair grooming routine and in the optimal hairstyles available to your curl type. Having a solid hair grooming routine is especially important in your quest to achieving an awesome mane, which is why knowing your curl type is of great use so as to fine-tune the needs of your curly mane. Conclusion? Make the effort to find out your curl type as per the instructions that you will find in the next subsection.

It must be said, however, that my proposed curl typing guide is neither absolute nor 100% bulletproof. It relies on finding out the vertical length that a full curl takes to form, which means that, for this specific measuring purpose, you will have to visualise your curly hair in 2 dimensions and not 3. This leaves some small margin for error that is already factored into the guide and for each of the curl types. When in doubt, repeat the measuring process and help the identifying process by using the examples of popular curly men that are referenced in each of the curl types. The goal is to measure the vertical length needed for your hair to form curls and then fit this worked-out vertical length into the proposed ranges of the guide so as to identify your curl type.

Efforts have been made in the past to classify hair into types, but none of the proposed guides have been successful in providing a solid, effective and conclusive typing option. I was inspired to create this guide during my awesome mane journey as I have had a large pool of men to test it on and because all the curly men I have talked with agreed that none of the current typing guides were of use to our curly hair as these guides were too abstract or didn't take into account that the majority of men carry their curls short, which makes typing men's hair more difficult than typing women's hair. My guide is approached from the novel and tested perspective that one's curls are predominantly formed within a range of vertical lengths, allowing us to classify our curls objectively instead of relying on subjective means as the rest of proposed guides do.

Since your curly hair is determined by your genes and the unique characteristics of your hair follicles, the vertical length needed to form curls as your hair grows is fairly uniform, thus your curls grow within a range of vertical lengths. This means that, for best typing results, your current curly hair should not have been altered prior to measuring; if your curly hair has been modified structurally via relaxers, texturisers, straightening irons or other straightening methods, your current curly hair will not represent your natural curl type. If you are part of the population of curly men who have altered their hair in such ways, it is then best that you wait until you outgrow your altered hair and sport your natural curls to then find out your curl type. In the meantime, you can work out an approximation of your curl type by looking at photos of yourself with your natural hair, and you can certainly continue to apply the rest of the knowledge that you will be acquiring with this book as you grow your new batch of an awesome mane.

Apart from any permanent structural modifications you may have done to your hair, the daily wear and tear of your hair can slightly alter the natural vertical length of your curls. This is unavoidable since trivial activities such as styling your hair or rubbing your head against the pillow during sleep can temporarily and slightly alter the natural vertical length of your curls. All of this is taken into account in the curl typing guide, and the only thing you should do prior to measuring your curls is to ensure that your hair is dry and not coated with hair products.

Finally, since each curl type is distinguished by how long it takes to vertically complete a curl, this typing guide doesn't include straight hair as straight hair doesn't curl. The cut-off mark for the vertical length dividing curly hair from straight hair is 3 inches as even straight hair in males will very slightly curve at a length of more than 3 inches from daily wear and tear. At the end of the day, however, straight hair can be managed for the most part as curly hair, so feel free to share all of the advice you will learn with your straight haired peeps or recommend this book to them. Unfortunately, the reverse is not true, and what works on straight hair will not work optimally on curly hair to yield an awesome mane, and thus the immense need for us curly males to acquire specific knowledge on our waves, coils and kinks.

Spotting a curl and knowing what it is

To identify your curl type, all you need is a ruler and knowing what it is that you are trying to measure.

Figure 3 – A curly haired lock

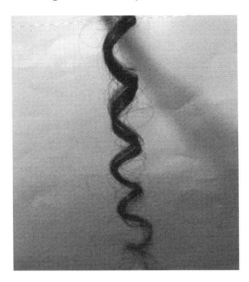

You will be aiming to measure the vertical length needed for a full curl to form in your hair. A curl occurs when the hair shaft is curving in one direction (clockwise) and then the direction is broken to start a new curve following the same clockwise direction of the preceding curve: the distance between the initial start of the curve (Point A) and the point where the direction of the curve breaks to start a new curve (Point B) is what forms a single full curl. Instead of measuring the distance of the curve itself in the hair shaft, however, what you want to measure is the vertical distance (i.e. shortest distance) between Point A and Point B (i.e. between the start of the curve and the end of the curve). Because curly haired strands have a tendency to group together as hair locks, instead of using a single hair strand, you will typically be using a hair lock to spot a full curl and measure its vertical length.

Now, take a few deep breaths. Read the above paragraph again. It may sound complicated at first, but, in reality, it is actually easy to spot and measure a full curl once you put yourself to the task. Ingrain in your mind what makes a curl and its vertical length, and then keep reading as the following paragraphs will fully expand on this curl-measuring concept. In the case that your hair is of such a kinky and tight nature that no hair locks are discernible, you can use a single hair strand instead to spot and measure a full curl.

Figure 4 – Illustration of what constitutes a full curl (A to B)

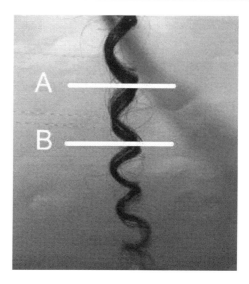

Spotting when a full curl occurs can be slightly tricky when you first give it a go, primarily because hair grows in 3 dimensions, not 2. As a curly haired lock continues to grow, the breaking of the curves' direction along the length of the lock leads to the formation of successive curls and a pseudo capital-E shape will be apparent as each curl leads on to the next. A full curl itself (Point A to B in Figure 4 above) resembles a C shape whereas 2 full curls, one following the other, resemble said E shape as shown next in Figure 5 with Curl 1 and Curl 2.

Figure 5 – Illustration of the E-shape effect from 2 full curls joining

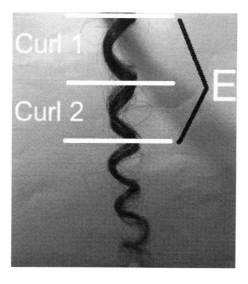

Once you identify a curl via its C shape, you will be able to see how the rest of the curls in the same lock lead from one another, forming E shapes throughout if the lock is long enough

as depicted in Figure 5. So long as you keep in mind these alphabetical cues of a full curl resembling a "C" and 2 full curls resembling an "E", you will be able to spot a full curl to measure. Next in Figure 6 is how a typical curly lock looks with its curls identified and ready to be measured:

Figure 6 – 4 full curls identified in a curly haired lock

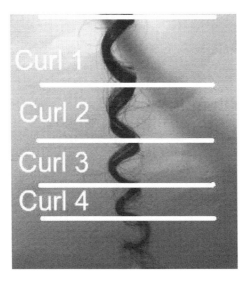

The lock of hair above is mine, and you can see how the curls blend into each other, with each full curl forming a C shape, and thus the E shapes forming as each curl in the lock follows from the previous one. Once the full curl has been identified, you will then proceed to measure its vertical length, which is the straight distance between the start of the curve and the breaking of the curve's direction (Point A to Point B as per Figure 4).

To further illustrate what the curl's vertical length encompasses, if we were to think of a full curl as a semicircle (i.e. a C shape), the length that would make the diameter of the semicircle would, in fact, be the length that is of interest to us and which needs to be measured. In the next diagram, you can see what a full curl would be with the C shape identified and how the C shape is visualised as a semicircle to measure its diameter (i.e. vertical length):

Figure 7 – The capital C letter

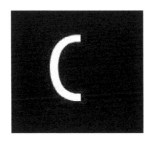

Figure 8 – A semicircle with its diameter shown (A to B)

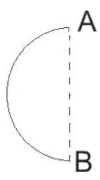

Going back to my own depicted lock in Figure 6 with the 4 curls identified, these are the vertical lengths that I measured for each of the curls:

- **Curl 1:** 0.9 inches (2.4 centimetres).

- **Curl 2:** 0.7 inches (1.9 centimetres).

- **Curl 3:** 0.7 inches (1.7 centimetres).

- **Curl 4:** 0.5 inches (1.3 centimetres).

As you can see above, the vertical length of each curl in my illustrated lock of hair is fairly uniform, differing by only a few millimetres (approximately 0.2 inches) except in the case of Curl 1, which differs by a few more millimetres and which has a reason behind it that I will explain a bit further down. For now, stay with the vertical lengths measured for Curl 2, Curl 3 and Curl 4.

The displayed uniformity in the curls' vertical lengths (i.e. minimal difference between curls) as each curl is formed in the hair lock is the commonality among all curly men because the curling of one's hair strands is determined genetically: the hair follicles in your scalp will continue to produce hair with the same determined curled vertical length on and on until you go bald and the follicles cease to produce any more hair material. Due to this uniformity in the vertical length of one's curls and it being the commonality among curly men, it is then feasible to rely on the measured vertical length of a curl to put one's curly hair into a type. Going back to my exemplified lock, the vertical lengths of all curls (including Curl 1) fall within the vertical length range for Type III curl type (0.5 – 1 inches). Ergo, I am a Type III curly haired male!

As emphasised in this subsection, the 2-dimensional C pattern formed by a single full curl is not always noticeable at first glance because curls do indeed grow in 3 dimensions and because one's curly hair may express itself as ringlets, springs, "Os", "Zs" and other peculiar forms of curves, twists and bends. However, if you bear in mind what a curl encompasses and that you are trying to measure the vertical length of the curl (shortest distance between Point A and Point B) and you also approach its visualisation and measurement in 2 dimensions, you will then be able to spot your curls for measurement.

Can you spot the curls in the following illustration (use the lock furthest to the right)?

Figure 9 – Example of several typical curly haired locks

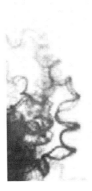

The curls in this illustration are expressed as coils just like mine, which can make the measurement of a given curl a slightly tricky thing. Some people would classify this curl type as "kinky" while others would call it "kinky-curly", and others would call it "coily", and some would simply say "curly" and leave it at that. However, if instead of guessing names, we actually measure the vertical length of the typical curl as explained and we do so with a 2-dimensional visualisation, we can then classify curly hair objectively. These are some of the curls that you should be able to spot on the lock that is furthest to the right by following the explained curl-measuring concept of our Curly Hair Type Guide:

Figure 10 – Full curls identified in a curly haired lock

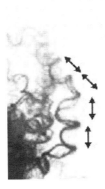

As mentioned earlier, and as illustrated with my example and this last example, the vertical length of each curl along a lock of hair remains fairly uniform, allowing us to fit the vertical length of our curls into any of the 5 available curl types.

You may, however, find out that you also seem to have another curl type expressing in your mane, yet this occurrence will be limited to specific parts of your scalp. Don't worry, this is perfectly normal, and you will have a curl type that is the predominant one out of the 2 curl types expressed. Most importantly, and as you will learn in the next subsection, the curls that are of relevance to measure are those found on the top of your head, not the sides or back of the head. To relate to my case, my curl type is a predominant Type III, but I also have Type IV curls in the nape and lower sides (close to the sideburns).

Following from the above, whenever one finds out that he has 2 curl types, the 2 types will be very similar and will be a number up or down from the predominant curl type. This slight discrepancy in one's curl type is most commonly noticed between the curls on the top of the head and the curls on the side and back of the head. The actual reason for this is because the hair on the back and sides of your head is constantly being pulled and rubbed against the pillow when you sleep. Considering that you spend about one quarter of your life laying on a bed, you can imagine the amount of beating that your curls get by just living your life! Lastly, the closer that scalp hair is to facial hair (e.g. sideburns and around ears), the tighter the curls tend to be as the scalp hair starts to resemble facial hair.

To illustrate the range of 5 curl types possible with curly hair, consider this: the loosest curl type of the 5 available (Type I) takes 2 to 3 inches to form a single full curl whereas the tightest curl type of the 5 available (Type V) takes a small fraction of an inch to form a single full curl. Such is the wild difference in vertical lengths required to form a full curl between curl types that, within the span of 3 inches, Type I curly hair will only form 1 full curl whereas Type V curly hair will form more than 10 full curls!

The following are the 5 types of curly hair available and the ranges of vertical lengths (imperial and metric) that each takes to form a full curl:

- **Type I:** 2 to 3 inches to form a full curl (5.1 centimetres to 7.6 centimetres).

- **Type II:** 1 to 2 inches to form a full curl (2.5 centimetres to 5.1 centimetres).

- **Type III:** 0.5 to 1 inch to form a full curl (1.3 centimetres to 2.5 centimetres).

- **Type IV:** 0.125 to 0.5 inches to form a full curl (0.3 centimetres to 1.3 centimetres).

- **Type V:** takes up to 0.125 inches to form a full curl (up to 0.3 centimetres).

As your curly hair grows, it forms curls at uniform vertical lengths falling under the range of one of the curl types above. It is the availability of these 5 vertical length ranges that makes all the curl types so disparate in looks and that yields their inherent hair grooming needs.

Working out the vertical length of your curly hair

Now that you know what a curl is and what is it that you are trying to measure, grab a ruler and get measuring. Before starting, make sure that your hair is fully dried and not coated with any hair products whatsoever as your goal is to measure the natural and genetically-programmed vertical length of your curly hair. For details on how to dry your hair, refer to the subsection on how to dry your curls in the next chapter.

Once you have ensured that your hair is ready for measurement, select a lock of hair from the top of your head; this is very important: only choose a lock of hair from the top of your head, not the sides or the back. This is because the top of your head is exposed the least to daily wear and tear, so the hair in this area yields the closest representation of what your true curl type is.

Figure 11 – Aerial view of top of the head & recommended area to select a lock of hair from

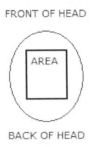

Grab a lock of hair from the area of the scalp shown in Figure 11 above, and gently lift the lock up while standing in front of a mirror so that you can see the chosen lock clearly. Now, place the ruler alongside the lock: you should place the ruler starting from the base of the lock if your hair is less than 6 inches in length; if you have hair longer than 6 inches, place the ruler starting from the tip of the lock instead.

Measure the vertical length of the first fully-formed curl. Do not exert any pulling tension on the hair lock, you want the lock to be gently held up so that you can spot the curl, that's all. When spotting the curl, think of the C-shape cue and use the first full curl formed starting from either the base or the end of the lock, depending on whether your hair length is under (start at base) or over (start at tip) 6 inches.

If your hair is long enough to have formed more than 1 full curl, aim to measure the second full curl formed instead of the first one formed, independent of whether you are measuring from the base or end of the lock. This is done because the first full curl in a lock of hair bears most of the weight of the lock itself if the hair is long enough to have formed more than 1 curl. On the other hand, the first full curl starting from the tip always takes the most beating when the hair is long enough to have formed more than 1 full curl. Consequently, measuring the second full curl formed, either from the base or tip, should be done when the lock has more than 1 full curl formed.

Once you have measured the vertical length of the given curl in your lock of hair, repeat the measuring process on 2 more locks close to the lock you have just measured (choose again from the same area of the scalp). There will be a slight natural variation between the vertical lengths recorded for your 3 locks; this is perfectly normal, so just work out the mean average of your 3 results, which will then give you the representative vertical length of your curly hair. Proceed to identify your curl type by matching your worked-out vertical length to any of the length ranges for each curl type. Here they are again:

- **Type I:** 2 to 3 inches to form a full curl (5.1 centimetres to 7.6 centimetres).

- **Type II:** 1 to 2 inches to form a full curl (2.5 centimetres to 5.1 centimetres).

- **Type III:** 0.5 to 1 inch to form a full curl (1.3 centimetres to 2.5 centimetres).

- **Type IV:** 0.125 to 0.5 inches to form a full curl (0.3 centimetres to 1.3 centimetres).

- **Type V:** takes up to 0.125 inches to form a full curl (up to 0.3 centimetres).

As curly hair can take up to 3 inches in vertical length to manifest a curl (e.g. Type I), you may find out that your current hair length doesn't allow for your hair to manifest a full curl yet. This occurs typically with short Type I or Type II curly hair; in such cases, you will be able to at least rule out those curl types that you will not be as you place the ruler alongside the lock and see that no full curl has formed at whatever length your hair is at the time. For example, if your hair is only 1 inch long in its natural state and no curl has formed by the 1-inch length mark, you would be able to rule out having Type III, IV and V curly hair and would only need to find out whether you have Type I or Type II curls. To then find out which of the 2 remaining curl types you have, you would either delay the measuring of the curl until you hair is a bit longer or you'd use the male references used for each curl type to make an educated guess.

Lastly, do you remember the measured curls in my lock of hair that I depicted earlier in Figure 6? The first fully-formed curl starting from the base of the lock (Curl 1) was a bit longer than the rest of the curls, and I told you that I would be explaining the reason for this. Here is the same lock with the 4 curls spotted:

Figure 12 – 4 full curls identified in a curly haired lock

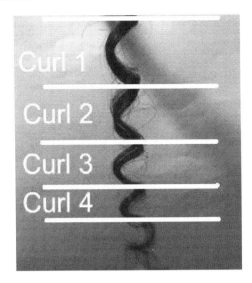

When curly hair has more than 1 fully-formed curl as is the case of my depicted lock above, the first full curl starting from the base of the lock bears the weight of the whole lock as well as any other form of tension applied on the hair, which means that the first full curl will not have a vertical length corresponding to its normal and genetically-determined vertical length. As you read in my example, Curl 1, with a vertical length of 0.9 inches or 2.4 centimetres, was bordering the upper vertical length range of Type III curly hair (the upper limit being 1 inch or 2.5 centimetres) whereas the rest of the curls had shorter, much more similar lengths.

In this depicted lock of mine, if I wanted to select a curl to measure, I'd be choosing Curl 2 as it is the second fully-formed curl starting from the base and the lock measures less than 6 inches in length. Moreover, take into account that in this lock I have measured the 4 curls only to help you visualise the spotting of curls in a lock of hair: you only need to measure 1 curl (starting from either the tip or base according to the lock's length), and you always measure a fully-formed curl.

That's the end of this subsection on how to work out the vertical length of your curly hair; that wasn't that bad, was it? Take the time to digest this subsection and understand the concept of the vertical length of your curly hair and the process of measuring it. Once you put all of this into practice, you will be able to see a side of your hair that you never thought would be possible and appreciate the usefulness of knowing your curl type.

Identifying your curl type: the 5 curl types

In this subsection, you can find all the 5 curl types described so that you can start getting used to your specific one. You can also find the 5 curl types expressed in a convenient table in Appendix XIV at the end of the book; the table contains each curl type with its main characteristics for quick reference.

Match your worked-out vertical length to any of the 5 vertical length ranges in the previous subsection to know your curl type, and then read more about your specific curl type below. From here henceforth, you will be applying any specific advice to your curl type, which will be mostly with regards to your hair grooming routine and the hairstyles suitable for your curl type. When in doubt about your curl type, even after repeatedly measuring your curls' vertical length, refer to the examples of popular men used for each curl type so as to help yourself in further defining the specific type of your hair.

Type I

Type I curly hair takes 2 to 3 inches of vertical length to form a single full curl. If your hair is shorter than 3 inches, you will be able to visibly notice your Type I curls curving at the 1.5-inch vertical-length mark. If your hair is shorter than 1.5 inches, compare your curls to those of the popular men referenced below and who also have Type I curly hair. This curl type is easy to mistake for straight hair at very short lengths, so it is important that you do identify it for what it is.

Type I curls tend to express themselves as waves, and this curl type is colloquially known as wavy hair or loose curls. Popular curly men with such curl type include Hugh Grant, George Clooney and Antonio Banderas.

Type II

Type II curls are the crunched version of the waves in Type I, and the vertical length required to form a full curl is shorter, from 1 inch to 2 inches. If your hair is shorter than 1 inch, you should be able to view a curved pattern already at the 0.5-inch vertical-length mark. Type II curly hair can be mistaken for straight hair at 0.25 inches in length and lower, so, if your hair is very short, do as for Type I curls and use the examples of popular men below if you hint that you have this curl type.

Type II curls form as a blend of waves and coils, and this curl type is colloquially known as tight waves, wavy hair or loose curls. Celebrities such as Adrian Grenier, Matthew McConaughey and Nick Jonas have Type II curls.

Type III

Type III curly hair takes 0.5 inches to 1 inch of vertical length to form a full curl. Type III curls will exhibit their curved pattern at a vertical length of 0.125 inches and will not be mistaken for straight hair at lower lengths. Due to the inherent shorter vertical length required to form Type III curls, this curl type quite commonly starts forming curls in a corkscrew and coiled pattern as opposed to the waves that Type I and II form. It doesn't matter, just approach their measurement in a 2-dimensional manner, and you will be able to measure their vertical length.

Type III curly hair is known colloquially as coils or ringlets, and it is the curl type of male celebrities such as Will Ferrell, Justin Timberlake and John Turturro.

Type IV

Type IV curly hair takes between 0.125 inches to 0.5 inches of vertical length to form a full curl. At any vertical length of less than 0.125 inches, the hair is curved and the curving pattern is easy to notice unless the hair is at a length equating a day's worth of stubble. Type IV curls are the crunched version of the coils in Type III curl hair; Type IV curls keep the coiled and spiral-like form of Type III curl, but Type IV curls are tighter by nature (i.e. Type IV curls form in a shorter vertical length).

Colloquially, Type IV is known as tight coils, kinky-curly or kinky hair, and examples of celebrities with such curl type include youngsters Corbin Bleu and Jaden Smith as well as NFL player Troy Polamalu.

Type V

Type V curly hair forms a full curl at near-shaved vertical lengths, from a day's worth of stubble all the way up to 0.125 inches of vertical length. This curl type expresses itself visibly as soon as it grows from the hair follicle, thus it is noticeable at cropped lengths. The main difference between Type IV curly hair and Type V curly hair is that Type V curly hair forms tight coils and kinks in the shortest vertical length of all curl types, hence the curl definition of this tightest curl type is hardly visible at first glance. This tightness of Type V curls poses a problem for getting very defined kinks, and, if you have this curl type, it is better that you don't worry about having the coiled definition of Type IV curls and instead concentrate on embracing the superb puffing-out nature of this curl type, which no other curl type has.

Type V curly hair is colloquially known as tight coils, kinky hair and, in some circles, as afro-textured hair. Type V is the curl type of popular curly men such as Cuba Gooding Jr, Will Smith and Morgan Freeman.

The next table (Figure 13) is the smaller version of Appendix XIII; Figure 13 illustrates all the curl types with their given characteristics. Keep this table in mind because as you move on to the hair grooming and hair care chapters, this table will start to become more and more relevant.

Figure 13 can be found in the Appendix as Appendix XIII and Appendix XIV. The shampooing and conditioning elements of the tables will be covered extensively in the next chapter.

Figure 13 – The 5 types of curly hair and their main characteristics

	CURLY HAIR TYPES				
	I	II	III	IV	V
Common name	Wavy	Wavy/Loose Curls	Coiled/Ringlets	Kinky/Kinky Curly	Kinky/Afro
Vertical Length of curl	2 to 3 inches	1 to 2 inches	0.5 to 1 inch	0.25 to 0.5 inches	-0.25 inches
Male references	Hugh Grant Antonio Banderas George Clooney	Adrian Grenier Matthew Mcconaughey Nick Jonas	Will Ferrell Justin Timberlake John Turturro	Corbin Bleu Jaden Smith Troy Polamalu	Cuba Gooding Jr. Will Smith Morgan Freeman
Shampooing frequency	Moderate	Moderate	Low	Low	Very low
Need for extra conditioning (normal + leave-in conditioner)	Low	Moderate	Moderate	High	High

The 2 lengths of hair

Hair can be measured in 2 states: fully extended and natural. Most commonly, when average Joes refer to the "length" of their hair, they refer to the length of hair measured when the hair has been pulled, flattened and extended. Rightfully so, however, you are reading these lines because you want to achieve an awesome mane, so thinking and knowing what average Joes do is not what we are here for; there is more to hair length than merely extending your curly locks and shouting numbers.

The hair length measured when the hair is pulled and fully extended is known as "extended length". On the other hand, the hair length measured when the hair is in its natural non-pulled state is known as "visible length". For what is worth, hair in males grows an average of 0.5 inches per month of extended length (stay with this important fact as it will soon become more relevant).

It is imperative for you to know your extended hair length as it relates highly to the grooming and caring approaches that you will use for your awesome mane. Visible hair length is not as relevant for your hair grooming or hair care, but it is especially useful to know in terms of considering hairstyles and for calculating how long your curls will take to reach lengths denoted by a certain body part (e.g. hair reaching shoulder length).

The 4 categories of extended hair length

The importance of knowing your extended hair length is due to the different necessities of curly hair at the different extended lengths it grows to, and you, as a curly haired male, must take into account this factor when approaching your awesome mane efforts.

In males, hair can be categorised in 4 extended lengths: near-shaved, short, medium and long. The difference between each is purely length related, and you would jump from one category to another as your hair grows or if you cut it. Extended length together with your curl type will define the grooming specifics of your awesome mane.

All other things equal, the longer your hair is, the more grooming efforts it will require from your part. Do not be put off by this, however, because even the longest of awesome manes can be fitted into a modern male's lifestyle so long as it is managed as an awesome mane and not as a dead rat. I, for example, can have my curls at a very long length (think Troy Polamalu) while spending less efforts and time than a typical curly dude would spend on his short curls. The trick? Well, that's what this book is all about!

These are the 4 categories of extended hair length for males:

Near-shaved

As the name implies, the hair has been cropped close to the scalp, and its visibility resembles that of stubble. This length does not allow for the formation of a full curl in any of the curl types except for Type V curly hair, and the length that the near-shaved category encompasses is from that of a day's worth of stubble up to 0.125 inches or from a #0 to a #1 in guard lengths in a hair clipper.

Short

This length goes from 0.125 inches up to 2 inches. It is a length that is chosen by many males with curly hair as it allows for the formation of full curls in most curl types and doesn't require much grooming or maintenance as opposed to the longer length categories. Only Type I curly hair will not exhibit a full curl at this length although, at the 2-inch mark, Type I curls will show a noticeable curving pattern.

Medium

This category ranges from 2 inches to 6 inches. Depending on your curl type, your curls will start to hang down (Type I or II) or they will still be standing up in a gravity-defying manner (Type III to V). Maintenance increases from that of a short length because the longer the curls grow, the more difficult it becomes for you to fully coat your curls with your own sebum, which increases your chances of having dry or unruly curls. Type III, IV and V will puff out at any medium length, and this inherent puffing out is a natural trait of these tighter curl types.

Long

This length goes from 6 inches and beyond. It is at this length that hair requires the most effort and maintenance from your part. In crude terms and sans any sugar coating, the longer your hair grows, the more the grooming and caring efforts involved because you will physically have more hair. Do not disregard this last sentence for I can assure you that you will be astonished at the amount of hair volume and physical mass that you have when you first grow your locks to 6 inches and beyond. Curly hair really is a double-edged sword as we naturally have far more hair volume than straight haired folks, but this trait has the potential to cause epic dead rats atop our heads. There is a reason for 99% of long haired dudes having straight hair!

Figure 14 – Inches of extended hair length per each hair length category

EXTENDED HAIR LENGTH	
Hair length (inches)	Hair length category
-0.125	Near-shaved
0.125 – 2	Short
2 – 6	Medium
6+	Long

Measuring the extended length of your hair

Just like with your curl type, you also want to get measuring here. This time, however, you will use a measuring tape, not a ruler, and you will measure you hair in its fully-extended state, not its relaxed and natural state. As opposed to gently holding up the hair lock like you did when measuring the vertical length of your curls, you will measure the extended length of your hair by gently pulling the lock until it is fully straightened and uncoiled (i.e. extended).

To measure your hair, ensure that your hair is dry and that you have a mirror and a measuring tape. You can use a ruler if you don't have access to a measuring tape, but I find the latter to be more convenient and useful for this task. Do the following:

- Stand in front of the mirror and identify the area of your scalp that has the largest collection of even-length hair strands; this will very likely be the top of your head. The purpose is to know the length that represents the majority of the hair strands in your scalp.

- Grab a lock of hair from this identified area of the scalp.

- Now, grab the measuring tape and pinch the start of the tape against the tip of the hair lock.

- Carefully and gently pull the tip of the hair lock so that the whole length of the lock is flattened and fully extended (i.e. no curving) as you simultaneously follow the measuring tape all the way down to the scalp (i.e. where the hair lock stems from).

- Make sure that the measuring tape is fully extended alongside the hair lock, do this by double-checking in the mirror. Grab the measuring tape at the point where it meets the base of the hair lock on the scalp.

- Record the length and repeat this process on 2 more hair locks next to the lock that you have recorded.

- Work out the mean average of the 3 results, and now match your hair length to any of the 4 extended length categories.

When you have worked out the extended length of your hair and the length category that it is in, write both results down and couple them with your curl type. Overall, while knowing your exact extended hair length is important, being aware of the length category of your hair is even more important so always know you current extended length category (i.e. near-shaved, short, medium or long) as it is essential for your hair grooming routine. Your curl type and your extended hair length category are 2 hair elements that will further define your awesome mane efforts and will become more and more relevant to you as you continue reading this book.

Visible hair length

Now that you know what extended hair length is and how to measure it, it is time to introduce to you the other hair length that is of relevance to us curly males: visible length. Visible hair length is the length that your hair has in its natural and non-extended state; in fact, you can think of visible hair length as the opposite of extended hair length.

Visible hair length is highly determined by your curl type because the tighter your curly hair is (i.e. shorter vertical length), the more it will be forming curls at a given length. To illustrate visible hair length and how it is affected by your particular curl type, think of yourself driving from Point A to Point B: imagine that you can choose to either take a straight road or a road with many bends and curves, which road starting at Point A would you choose to get the fastest to Point B? Of course, you'd choose the straight road or at least the one with less bends and curves. With visible length and curl type, it is very much like this: the tighter the curl type (i.e. more bends), the longer it will take to reach a determined visible length.

Figure 15 – A straight line (A to B) vs. a curved line (A to B)

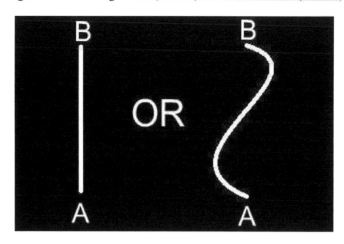

While extended length and its category are of extreme relevance to your hair grooming and hair care, visible length is of value to specifically know how long it will take you to achieve a determined length or even hairstyle. For example, a typical male's distance from the top of the head to the base of the neck is about 12 inches (this can vary by a few inches in men so do not panic if your distance is only 9 inches!). This means that for someone with straight hair (think a straight road), it'd take him exactly 24 months to have the hair on top of his head cover the 12 inches needed to reach the base of his neck (at a hair growth rate of 0.5 inches per month). Of course, a curly dude such as yourself cannot relate to the growth timespan of someone with straight hair because your hair will naturally take the longer path and curve and bend on its way.

Let's apply the above example to a curly haired male wanting to grow the 12 inches of visible length needed for his curls to reach the base of the neck: starting from a shaved length on the top of the head, a male with Type I curly hair would take about 30 months and a male with Type V curly hair would take 72 months (that's 6 years for Type V!).

Remember how at the beginning of this section I asked you to stay with the fact that the 0.5 inches of hair growth in males was of extended length? Indeed, this 0.5 inches of extended length is shortened as our waves, coils and kinks curve and bend as they grow from the hair follicle, yielding a much lower rate of "visible" hair growth than the 0.5 inches that the hair has factually grown in 1 month, and thus the reason for curly haired men (and women) always complaining about how their hair takes so long to grow. In other words, while the straight haired folks are getting a full 0.5 inches of visible length every month due to their naturally-straightened hair strands, we curly folks only get a fraction of that 0.5 inches in visible length in that same timespan. Literally, a dude with Type V curls will have to wait 3 times more than a straight haired dude to get his curls to the same visible length. Curly hair dramas, anyone?

Bearing in mind all of the above and the differences between extended and visible length, I have created a very useful table (Figure 16 below) that will allow you to have a guideline as to how long it will take your hair to look like (i.e. visible length) starting from a fully-shaved length.

Figure 16 – Timespans needed to grow each curl type to each visible hair length (months)

	VISIBLE HAIR LENGTH				
	Shaved	2 inches	4 inches	6 inches	12 inches
Straight hair	0	4	8	12	24
Type I	0	5	10	15	30
Type II	0	6	12	18	36
Type III	0	8	16	24	48
Type IV	0	10	20	30	60
Type V	0	12	24	36	72

The time it will take you to achieve a certain visible length may differ by a few months, but I would highly recommend you to go by the timespans in the table above (Figure 16) as I have found them to be precise on myself and on other curly males I have tested it on. This means that if you have, say, Type IV curly hair and you want to sport a shoulder-length hairstyle (base of the neck, 12 inches of visible length required), you should give yourself at least 60 months to get there if you are growing your hair from a shaved-hair length.

By all means, play around with the numbers if you have other current visible hair lengths. All you have to do is subtract the month number in your current visible length from the month number in the new visible length that you want to achieve, the difference will be the time it will take you to get to that desired visible length.

Another example, let's assume that your curls are currently bordering 4 inches in visible length and you are a Type III wanting to grow to a visible 6 inches of hair length. If you look at the table above, you will see that the 6-inch visible length mark requires approximately 24 months to grow from a shaved length. Simply subtract the months of your current visible length (16 months for your current 4 inches of visible length) from these 24 months, and you will find out that it will take about 8 months to grow the 2 inches of visible length needed to get from your current 4 inches of visible length to your desired 6 inches of visible length.

If your visible hair length is not any of the 5 visible lengths in the table (shaved, 2, 4, 6 or 12 inches), I recommend you to round your current visible hair length down to any of those 5 lengths and not round up. For example, if your current visible hair length is 3.5 inches and you want to find out how long it will take you to reach 12 inches, use the number of months in the 2-inch length column and not the 4-inch length column. This is because when estimating hair growth timespans, you should always be conservative and expect the longest time rather than the shortest time.

To measure your current visible length, you should do exactly as you'll do for your extended length. The only difference will be that you will not pull the hair lock to straighten it; rather, you will measure the lock in its natural state without any pulling or modifying, ensuring that you measure the length between the base of the lock and its tip without bending the ruler or measuring tape. Likewise, you must measure the visible length when your hair is fully dried and not coated with any hair products whatsoever. The best way to go about this is by soaking your hair in the morning, not applying any hair products (e.g. no hair gel) and then going about your day as the hair dries on its own. Once you see that the hair has dried completely, proceed to measure your visible length.

Know your hair lengths

Take your time to absorb and digest what you have read on hair lengths. Read a few times what extended and visible lengths are, understand their differences and obtain each one of them, remembering that knowing your current extended hair length category is crucial for your hair grooming and hair care. Work out your 2 hair lengths and pair them together with your curl type. Are you a long haired (10 inches) Type III or are you a Type V with short curls? How about having loose curls, are yours specifically a Type I or a Type II, and what actual extended and visible lengths are they? If you have Type IV curls at 2 inches of visible length, how long would it take you to get them to a visible length of 6 inches?

In addition to knowing your hair lengths, I have also created a table (Figure 17, after this paragraph) that will allow you to estimate the approximate extended length that you will have at whichever visible hair length you have. This table will allow you to calculate your future extended length category when you grow your hair to a certain visible length. Since your extended hair length category is what matters for your hair grooming and hair care efforts, you can then anticipate any changes to the physical part of your awesome mane that are dependent on your extended hair length category.

Figure 17 – Estimation of extended hair length at each visible hair length (inches)

	VISIBLE HAIR LENGTH				
	Shaved	2 inches	4 inches	6 inches	12 inches
Straight hair	0	2	4	6	12
Type I	0	2.5	5	7.5	15
Type II	0	3	6	9	18
Type III	0	4	8	12	24
Type IV	0	5	10	15	30
Type V	0	6	12	18	36

Visible hair length is useful because it will allow you to work out your hair growth timespans, but it is the extended hair length and its category that matter for your hair grooming and hair care. Do note that from here onwards, any mentions of "hair length" or "length" as a generic term will be referring to extended length and not visible length. If at any time I want to refer to visible length, I will do so by using the specific term itself (i.e. visible length).

Other interesting tidbits you can know about your curly hair

Your curl type, your extended hair length category and your 2 hair lengths are the 4 most important elements to know prior to moving on to achieve and master your awesome mane. Knowing these elements will be the first step in your awesome mane journey, and they will inherently provide an instant boost to said journey, putting you in a position to start taking further steps and actions. Likewise, these 4 elements are the preludes to your hair knowledge, and they will enhance your learning as you continue advancing in this book. Thus, make the effort to know your curl type, your 2 hair lengths and your extended hair length category before doing anything else concerning your awesome mane.

There are other hair elements that play a minor role in your awesome mane and that are worth the mention if anything so that you can relate even more to the advice that you will be encountering in the following chapters. An awesome mane works greatly when approached from the Pareto principle in that 80% of results can be achieved with 20% of the effort needed to achieve 100% results, only that, in the case of an awesome mane, the 20% of effort that matters will bring 95% results instead of 80% of results. In other words, take home the message of knowing your curl type, your 2 hair lengths and your extended hair length category, but also be aware of the following hair tidbits:

Hair density

This refers to how many hair strands you have per square centimetre. Many people have a mistaken idea of what hair density is and erroneously use the term "dense hair" to refer to hair that looks big or is long. Losing hair density is the main effect of going bald (male pattern baldness) as the number of hair strands in a given square centimetre is reduced gradually until there are no more hair strands growing from the follicles (i.e. baldness). Your hair density is determined by your genes, and blonde people tend to have the highest density whereas black haired and red haired people have the lowest. The higher the hair density you have, the harder your hair will be to style and the higher the potential for your hair to look voluminous.

Hair thickness

This refers to how thick an individual hair strand is, or, in other words, it refers to the cross-sectional circumference of the hair shaft. "Thick hair" is also erroneously used by most people to describe hair that looks bushy or voluminous. You can easily have voluminous bushy-looking hair but at the same time have thin hair strands, and, just like with hair density, hair thickness is determined by our genes. Hair thickness becomes a bit more relevant when your hair reaches a long length and you want it to hang down fully.

Coil factor

This refers to the difference between your extended hair length and your visible hair length. The coil factor is the main reason behind curly men complaining about how they never have enough hair length and how their hair never seems to hang down. Essentially, hair is growing at all times, but, due to the curving pattern of curly hair, visible hair growth takes very long to manifest, and, at short lengths, all curl types have a tendency to puff out instead of to hang down. The coil factor becomes more prominent and noticeable the tighter the curls are, and it is one of those things that you just have to live with and embrace.

Damp vs. Dry (DvD)

This is the visual difference between how your hair looks when it is damp (e.g. after a shower) and how it looks when it dries fully (e.g. a few hours after a shower). It has to do with your coil factor as the hair strands are weighted down and extended in length when the hair is damp; once the hair fully dries, the curls return to their natural state and visible length, unless limited by whatever hair products the hair strands may be coated with. Since I will be using the DvD effect a few times in this book, let me take this opportunity to remind you that "damp" refers to when your hair is lightly covered in water and is not soaked or dripping water: this wetness state is normally achieved by removing the excess water with a towel or by shaking your head back and forth and to the sides. Damp is the wetness state that you should style your curls in (styling will be covered in the next chapter).

Accumulated hair damage

This hair element is important to have mentioned because damaged hair will be hair that is unresponsive to awesome mane actions. The hair shaft doesn't have an intrinsic ability to repair itself, which is why you should treat your hair carefully. I always tell men to treat their hair as they'd treat their car: if you bump your car and damage the chassis, you can take it to the mechanic and get it fixed, but the chassis will never look and feel as a brand-new chassis. Luckily, you can outgrow the damaged hair, but the process can be very lengthy, so better be safe than sorry and strive to manage your curls on a daily basis with the hair care measures that you will learn in the fourth chapter.

As I have covered already in this chapter, if your current hair has been damaged (i.e. it has been relaxed, straightened or dyed), your best move to start owning an awesome mane is to cut your hair and grow a new batch of hair. Hair can be damaged easily even when manipulating it to put it into a hairstyle, and one of the reasons for failing to obtain an awesome mane is having damaged hair. Furthermore, and as I have emphasised throughout this chapter, hair is continuously growing, so don't be put off by cutting your hair, it will grow back in place!

Advantages and disadvantages of curly hair

Unfortunately, badly managed curly hair gives a lot of problems. You and I know that very well, and it took me years to finally turn my beast into a Labrador dog. With that said, an awesome mane will be very docile, and many of the hair dramas that you had before will be wiped out with an awesome mane.

As with anything you have in life, curly hair has its advantages and disadvantages. It is not my style to whine about how bad curly hair is or how unlucky we are to be curly haired: the attitude to achieve an awesome mane implies leaving behind all defeating tones, whining and cry-babying that we all curly haired dudes have done at one point or another as we have become tired of our beasts and dead rats. With your awesome mane, you will be able to maximise the advantages of your curly hair while taming the disadvantages, that simple. However, I am not here to paint the picture for you as colourful rainbows and happy unicorns either, and I want you to be realistic and be aware of those aspects, negative and positive, that our hair texture has by default.

Let's start first with the disadvantages of curly hair, so the advantages sound even better when you read them!

Disadvantages:

- Predisposition to dryness: this is the main issue with curly hair. Sebum is spread with difficulty through the hair haft with all the curves and bends of our texture, meaning that the vast majority of curly dudes walk around with hair that is not properly sebuminised, which in turn causes dryness and the feared dead rat effect. Since sebum protects our waves, coils and kinks, dry non-sebuminised hair becomes brittle, frizzes and looks dim. Dry hair is the biggest enemy that you will be facing in your daily awesome mane endeavours.

- Easy to be damaged: due to the curving nature of the hair strands, the shaft in curly hair doesn't have a uniform tensile strength across its length. This makes curly hair prone to being damaged when manipulated and enhances the need for getting the secreted sebum (plus conditioning products) coating the curls as much as possible while avoiding any unnecessary tension on the hair strands.

- Tangling: I always laughed it off when I heard my girlfriends complaining about their tangled hair. Then, I grew my beast to a mere 4 inches for the first time, and I was hit hard with the tangling, which got me understanding what a hair drama was. Due to the inherent curvylicious nature of our curly hair, our locks have a tendency to grab to each other and tangle, mat and knot. How much of it does it occur? It depends on the individual, but, as a rule of thumb, the higher your curl type and the longer your hair, the higher the risk of experiencing tangles and the likes. And yes, you have just read the word "curvylicious" in this paragraph.

- Doing whatever it wants: as you quite likely know already, curly hair seems to have a life of its own. One day you wake up, and your hair looks awesome; the next day, it's a huge mess, and you just feel like shaving it all. Likewise, you style your curls in an uber-cool hairstyle, and, 4 hours later, your hair looks like a mesh of who-knows-what. This is an issue shared among all curly haired men, and it is why many of us can't be bothered to try to do something about our own curls and thus the popularity of buzz cuts. Fortunately, one of the cool aspects of achieving an awesome mane is that you get to control how your curly hair looks and acts as you optimise your hair grooming and hair care.

- Difficult to style: this ties in with the above. Pulling your hair, being limited in hairstyles and not knowing what to do with your hair are the bread and butter for those men who don't own an awesome mane. As you will be learning, you need to throw away your pocket comb, get your fingers involved and know what you can and cannot do in terms of hairstyles.

- Difficult to grow: I am willing to bet that the thought of growing your curls long has crossed your mind at one point or another. However, since your curls take a lot of effort to manage at even medium lengths, you will very likely have crossed off the idea of growing your locks after imagining the enduring dramas and pain that growing your hair would entail. There's no denying it, curly hair is more difficult to grow than straight hair, and, generally, the higher your curl type, the more challenging the hair-growing journey becomes. Not all is lost, however, as I've had my awesome mane at a length reaching my navel, and the time I spent grooming it was minimal enough to fit it into a professional career and a modern lifestyle. The trick? An awesome mane itself: having an awesome mane means that you will dramatically cut down your bathroom time regardless of your curl type and hair length.

- Prejudice: this one is mild but is worth the mention. Having curly hair is seen, by some people, as funny, rebellious or different. This is stupid and stems from people having insecurity issues themselves. When I say people, I say men, for it is only those men with an inferiority complex or with serious insecurity issues who make comments or point at one for having curly hair. There is nothing wrong with being different, and there is certainly nothing wrong with embracing that which is inherent to you, whether it is your hair, skin, lifestyle or whatever it is that makes you different and unique. Moreover, properly groomed and looked-after curly hair (i.e. an awesome mane) will prevent any of this stupidity happening in the first place, and an awesome mane will also improve your self-confidence and image. Remember, an awesome mane is carried assertively and requires an attitude that will merely cause you to feel pity for the seldom few who try to discriminate you for having curly hair.

That's 7 disadvantages to curly hair right there; they seem like a lot, huh? Curly hair is a beast on its own, but it too has its benefits, which far outweigh any of its disadvantages. Check them out:

Advantages:

- <u>Volume:</u> because of its bends and curves, curly hair always looks bigger than it really is. You will never lack volume, and your hair will be visible to anyone from miles away. This volumising ability is especially useful for those balding curly men as it will make the balding less noticeable. About 65% of men are balding profusely by age 60, so at least you know that you will still have a decent mane in your old age to impress the nurses with when you go for your monthly doctor appointments!

- <u>Spices up your head:</u> because of the different curl types available, this hair variety gives you a more unique image to build yourself with. Every man with curly hair looks different, and since a properly looked-after set of curls on a male is very rare, an awesome mane will instantly make you stand out in any situation and have you subconsciously communicating to others that boosted confidence in yourself. Ever heard the phrase "don't mess with a curly haired man"? What, you haven't? Well, you are about to start making it popular, then.

- <u>Curly hair is sexy:</u> of course, we are talking about awesome-mane-type curls. One of the first things I noticed when I achieved my awesome mane was that women thought my hair was sexy, and they would actually tell me so in my face! Don't underestimate the sexiness of an awesome mane, I can assure you that you will never look back to your dead rat and buzz cut days.

- <u>It looks masculine:</u> due to its rebellious and big-volume nature, curly hair exudes self-confidence and manliness when it is looked after properly. As soon as you walk into a room, the first thing people will see on you is your hair; it enhances your presence and shows that, if you have the guts to own a beast like that and risk having it do whatever it wants (remember the previous disadvantages?), you are willing to take your chances on anything that is put in front of you. You carry your curly hair with pride because you have the guts to address your problems, fix them and turn weaknesses into strengths. And that's what real men do.

As I have said before, an awesome mane will tame all those disadvantages and maximise the advantages. Many of the men whom I have helped over the years have emphasised how much better they looked and felt with themselves, and how much more attention they received from women. Boosted self-confidence was always one of the benefits these awesome-mane men experienced, and all it took them was swapping their dead rats and buzz cuts for awesome manes. With knowledge comes the mane and the awesomeness, my friend.

My personal experience

Before venturing into experimenting with my hair, I knew I needed to know the basics of it. I have studied the biology of hair, consulted hairdressers and barbers, gone through cosmetology resources, delved into online databases designed for medical students and bugged those family members of mine who are in the medical field with questions on everything to do with the biological side of hair. I believe in experimentation but only after having educated oneself, otherwise one will be doomed for failure. I regard my success in achieving an awesome mane and helping others achieve theirs too as the result of learning as much as I could while always aiming to understand the actual mechanism of all actions I would implement, not just their consequences. If something failed, I would go back to the drawing board, and I would seek a better and improved action to implement.

Hair gets a lot of attention because humans recognise each other via their faces, and hair just happens to sit on top of the head, so it is only normal that we humans put a lot of effort into modifying our hair and making it look its best. Hair also has a strong evolutionary reason as, back in our caveman days, it was a useful cue to decide whether we wanted to mate with someone or not. Coincidentally, ask any woman these days what physical traits they seek in their perfect man, and "good hair" comes at the top of the list. While we have evolved socially and have swapped our caves for comfy condos, it is a reality that we still retain much of the brain of our primitive ancestors.

Acquiring my awesome mane led to a boost in my self-confidence as I knew that the stuff atop my head was now under my control. By default, I also looked better, and I noticed an interesting occurrence with the opposite sex: many times, it would be them, not me, breaking the ice to flirt with me by using the excuse of enquiring about my curly hair and going as far as calling my curls "luscious", "luxuriant" or "curvylicious". I am talking about ladies approaching me in the supermarket, gym or in the street, and plenty of guys have reported back to me of having the same occurring to them once they got their awesome manes. I will talk about this interesting benefit a bit more in the chapter dedicated to the mental part of an awesome mane, but I will tell you right now that I am not the sexiest man on the planet. Women genuinely love a well-groomed curly mane and the confidence in oneself that an awesome mane exudes; it ain't called "awesome" for no reason!

You know the cliché, with knowledge comes power, and that's precisely what you need for your awesome mane. It should not be too complicated, though, and I have always strived to approach hair from a convenient and modern-male angle. I have, however, overdone the whole hair-knowing aspect because I was determined to really get to know everything I could of my hair. Of course, this implied experimenting with my hair, and off I went with doing all sort of stuff to my hair. Overall, I found that a positive attitude plus a solid hair grooming routine and an optimal hair care strategy was all it took to really get my curls looking awesome.

In terms of the foundation of my hair knowledge, the most important part to my awesome mane has been knowing my curl type and knowing at what extended and visible lengths my hair was at in any given moment. And while it took me years to acquire, polish and perfect the knowledge that I am giving you with this book, I have always strived to prioritise the modern-male perspective in all of my hair-hacking matters; you and I have other things to do and achieve in our lives outside that of an awesome mane.

The next chapter is about hair grooming, so make sure that you have grasped this chapter fully because both these chapters are strongly related and I will be referencing much of the content of this 101 chapter. Furthermore, the way in which you go about your hair grooming will make or break your awesome mane, so you really want to ensure that you make the most of the next chapter!

3) Hair Grooming: Get Those Curls Looking Great

"Daily practice is essential to the achievement of any real success"

Arthur Saxon

Hair grooming refers to the daily process of making your curls look the part, and it is composed of 3 sequential stages: cleaning, conditioning and styling. Due to the manner in which the 3 stages complement each other, you should regard hair grooming as a routine and as an essential and integral aspect of your awesome mane. In other words, your hair grooming routine is what makes or breaks your awesome mane.

Most curly men are clueless when it comes to grooming their curls, and it is not their fault. The hair grooming industry is driven by a straight-hair focus because straight hair is much easier to manage and behave than curly hair: straight hair looks great in photo shoots and is the best texture for modelling a hairstyle. Hair grooming for men is already limited as it is, and, since most of the hair grooming information going around is only applicable to those with straight hair, men with curly hair find themselves with little to no relevant information for their manes. I mean, all these hair experts need to do is to try and do a Side Swept hairstyle on someone with Type IV curls to see how irrelevant their advice is to a good percentage of the world's male population!

Hair grooming is performed every day and starts from the moment that you jump in the shower: you start the routine by first cleaning the hair with either a shampoo or your fingers, then continue by coating the hair with a conditioner, and you finish your mane's grooming matters by styling the hair. The next step? You leave your house with an awesome mane that you are proud to be carrying on top of your head.

To put it bluntly, optimal hair grooming is what takes an average curly mane from a mess of unruly curly locks to a great-looking head of curls that enhance the image and self-confidence of its owner. What's more is that you don't need to be spending half of your day in the bathroom to get your hair rocking or have to share your lady's pile of hair products. In fact, one of the awesome parts of an awesome mane is that you get to carry your beast looking as desired in a convenient and non-girly manner; I have been doing that for quite a few years, so it is indeed possible!

Ok, so now that I have stressed to you the importance of hair grooming, you need to know what you will need for the magic to happen, which in essence boils down to a shampoo, your fingers, a conditioner, a hairstyle idea and a hairstyling product. The steps to implementing your hair grooming are as follows:

1) Jump in the shower.

2) Use a shampoo or your fingers to clean your hair.

3) Rinse the shampoo.

4) Apply the conditioner to the hair.

5) Rinse the conditioner and get out of the shower.

6) Use some hairstyling product to put your curls into a hairstyle.

7) Leave the bathroom and face the day with an awesome mane.

Not bad, isn't it? The above is the template of the hair grooming routine that you will be using for your curls and that I will cover in depth in this chapter. There's no need to make it fancy and hard to implement, a basic template with a few tweaks according to your individual needs is all you will need for your awesome mane. As basic as it may seem, your hair grooming routine can be a bit tricky initially to master, but the more you practise it, the better you will get at it. Just like anything in life, really.

If you were to try and dig into the semantics of the above routine, you would be able to quickly see that the stages of our hair grooming routine consists of 3 main actions:

- Cleaning (i.e. first stage)

- Conditioning (i.e. second stage)

- Styling (i.e. third stage)

To clean the hair, you use a shampoo or your fingers; to give your hair optimal gloss and smoothness, you use a conditioner; to style your curls, you must have a hairstyle idea and a hairstyling product to make it possible. Moreover, and as you will be learning later on, cleaning your hair with your fingers in the first stage is quite a valid approach; I have termed this approach the Sebum Coating method, and, as it relates to your hair grooming routine, every day you have to choose whether to use a shampoo or your fingers (i.e. Sebum Coating method) to clean your hair, with this decision being based upon your tailored shampooing frequency: there will be days in which you will shampoo your hair and other days in which you will instead use the Sebum Coating method to clean your hair.

The 3 hair grooming stages (i.e. cleaning, conditioning and styling) make the sequence and backbone of your hair grooming routine, and each stage has a main action and subsequent secondary actions. Furthermore, the backbone of the stages and their main actions remains unaltered in all days, but the secondary actions do change according to the day. For example, while the first stage in your hair grooming has a main action of cleaning the hair, both shampooing and the Sebum Coating method are 2 secondary actions as both are options available to perform the cleaning action (hence their "secondary" denomination), and these 2 secondary actions are exchanged according to the given day. Other secondary actions include conditioning your hair or using the Sebum Coating method to also condition your hair (second stage), or putting your hair into a hairstyle to style your hair (third stage).

Figure 18 – Hair-grooming main actions and their respective secondary actions

STAGES	SECONDARY ACTIONS			
Cleaning	Shampooing	Sebum Coating method		
Conditioning	Use normal conditioner	Sebum Coating method	Skip conditioning	
Styling	Use leave-in conditioner	Use hairstyling agent/s	Put hair into hairstyle	Dry hair

In this chapter, you will be learning all about the above, so for now just stay with the fact that your hair grooming routine is made up of 3 stages that imply 3 main actions: cleaning (first stage), conditioning (second stage) and styling (third stage). The 3 stages are carried out in the same sequence in every single day of the life of your awesome mane, but the choice of secondary actions is subject to daily variations. Having all of this worked out and put on autopilot is what will totally revamp your curly hair, hence the need for you to have a routine that supports an orderly and methodical grooming of your to-be-acquired awesome mane.

First stage – Cleaning

Cleaning your hair is the first stage of your hair grooming routine. When it comes to cleaning one's hair, most people think of using a shampoo. Indeed, shampoos are the best-known tools to clean your hair, but there is another form of cleaning your hair that you will be using on some days to substitute the shampoo; I have coined it the Sebum Coating method, and it involves the use of your fingers to clean the hair via the running of your fingers along the hair locks to create mechanical friction.

The problem with shampooing is that shampoos are very powerful hair-cleaning agents and using them daily is counterproductive because shampoos remove the much-needed sebum from the hair strands, which ultimately creates an instant dead rat if the shampoo is used too frequently or too much. The trick lies in scheduling shampooing days every so often and then using the Sebum Coating method to clean the hair on those days that no shampoo is used. What's more is that the Sebum Coating method not only cleans the hair but also helps to spread the secreted sebum along the hair strands, thus the Sebum Coating method has a strong conditioning action too.

Your hair grooming routine will be built around your worked-out shampooing frequency. Because shampoos are so powerful, you will need to use a hair conditioner following the rinsing of the shampoo to restore the gloss of your hair. On those days that you don't shampoo, you will have the option of skipping the hair conditioner for your second stage and instead satisfy your second stage with the Sebum Coating method due to this method's dual cleaning and conditioning actions.

In summary, you will start your hair grooming routine every day by either shampooing your hair or doing the Sebum Coating method, and, once you have finished implementing either of these 2 secondary actions for your cleaning stage, you will move on to the second conditioning stage.

Shampooing

Shampooing is a secondary action and is typically performed when you jump in the shower and soak your hair in water. Once soaked, the hair is cleaned with a shampoo, and the shampoo is then rinsed to finalise the cleaning stage.

Shampoos are mild detergents designed to remove (i.e. clean) any residue, grease or dirt from your hair. Shampoos contain specific blends of ingredients in their formulations that carry out the purported cleaning action; most commonly, a blend of sulfate-type ingredients is used in the formulation. Shampoos are effective at doing their job, but, in doing so, they strip away the precious scalp sebum that we curly dudes need to keep our manes looking our best.

There is a widespread belief that one must shampoo daily; this is not only wrong, but it is also counterproductive to men with curly hair desiring to sport an awesome mane. Curly hair has enough of a problem getting coated with one's own sebum, and shampoos completely kill the process of optimally coating the hair strands with sebum. Remember, shampoos act as detergents, so they will strip away everything, from the bad to the good; this is why you, as a curly haired male, should pay attention to how you go about using shampoo and need to find out an optimal shampooing frequency that has you using shampoo every X number of days.

On top of most curly men shampooing too frequently (i.e. daily), we add more insult to our manes by using too much shampoo every time that we use this hair-cleaning product: a "less is more" attitude should be used with shampoos. What's just as bad is that lather, which men associate with better shampooing results, is a double-edged sword, and men with curly hair have a tendency to create way too much lather as they shampoo. Instead, you should create as little lather as possible and strive to concentrate the shampoo and lather on the scalp, not along the length of the hair strands.

Using shampoo correctly as part of your hair grooming routine for an awesome mane is key, yet it can also be a bit awkward to manage in the beginning; you will soon become efficient at shampooing though, and it will become instinctive. It will pay off great awesome-mane dividends to learn how to use shampoos optimally, so do put in the effort because the end results will astonish you.

The optimal shampooing method

To optimally shampoo your awesome mane, you must follow these steps:

1) Soak all of your hair in water.

2) Grab the shampoo bottle and squeeze out a fingertip amount of shampoo, enough to cover the tip of your index finger.

3) Place the squeezed-out fingertip of shampoo on the centre of the top of your head.

4) Repeat Step 2 and Step 3, but instead of placing the squeezed-out shampoo on the centre of the top your head, place each fingertip amount on the following 5 more segments of your head (squeeze out a fingertip for every segment):

   a. The centre of the forehead's hairline (front of the top of the head).

   b. Each side of the head, right above the ears.

   c. The centre of the vertex area (back of the top of the head).

   d. The area located 4 inches above the nape (back of the head at about ear level).

5) Once you complete Step 4, use the tips of your index, middle and ring fingers (joined as if making a pad) to gently massage each segment of the scalp where the shampoo rests, aiming to spread the shampoo evenly in a 4-inch radius. Do this:

   a. Work on 2 segments at a time, using each hand for each segment (remember to use the 3 fingertips making a pad).

   b. Pair the segments so as to massage them simultaneously as follows: forehead & vertex, centre of top of head & nape, and the 2 sides of the head; start in that order too.

   c. Spend 20 seconds on the paired segments and massage in a circular motion. Do not use running water as you massage; when shampooing, running water is only used to either soak your hair or to rinse the shampoo.

6) Allow the lather created in Step 5 to sit naturally on the scalp. Do not spread it any further than what has been created by the massaging motion. It is fine if some lather unintentionally covers parts of your hair locks, just don't actively promote the coating of your curls with lather. You want the lather to be sitting primarily on the scalp; that is, on the surface of your head's skin.

7) Once you have finished massaging the last paired segments (i.e. sides of head), use running water from the shower bulb to rinse the shampoo. Tilt your head forward or backward so that the lather is washed away effectively and without getting in your eyes.

That is it. Even when pressed for time, this shampooing method will fit in nicely in anyone's busy schedule as the most that it will take is 5 minutes, and that's being uber conservative with the time. As you learn to master the above method, you will progressively cut down the time that it takes you to implement your shampooing.

The massaging of your scalp with the shampoo will take you just 1 minute since you will be massaging 2 segments at a time for a count of 20 seconds, the complete soaking of your hair will take you 30 seconds, the messing around with placing the shampoo on your scalp will take you another 60 seconds, and the rinsing of the shampoo will take you 30 seconds (if at all). You can realistically cut down the whole shampooing process to 3 minutes once you get good at it, and you will get good at it in a short timespan once you get practising.

The main thing to remember is that you want the shampoo to do most of its work on the scalp, not along the full length of the hair strands. As curly men, one of our biggest problems when it comes to our manes is that our secreted sebum tends to accumulate excessively on the scalp and on the base of the hair shaft, leaving the rest of the hair shaft, from mid-length to the tip, with little sebum coating, and thus the cause for dryness and brittleness commonly found in curly hair. You do not want the shampoo to be doing much of its job close to the ends of your hair; instead, you want the shampoo to clean your scalp and remove any excessive sebum accumulation on the segment of the shaft closest to the scalp. This same issue of overaccumulation occurs with hair products too; they have a tendency to accumulate on the base of the hair shaft especially if applied incorrectly, which makes the use of hair products as part of the styling stage a tricky thing.

Shampoos are powerful cleaning agents, so bear that in mind when using them as improperly-used shampoo will dry out your moisturised and sebuminised curls in an instant. In fact, one of the main causes for a dead rat is precisely using too much shampoo and thus continually robbing one's locks from the much-needed scalp sebum!

The optimal shampooing frequency

Now that you know the optimal shampooing method, it is time to learn how to find out your optimal shampooing frequency, which is just as important as how you go about applying the shampoo. Your shampooing frequency is central to your hair grooming routine, and the rest of secondary actions in all stages of your hair grooming routine will be dependent on your shampooing frequency.

As you know, shampoos are great at stripping away everything from your hair, including your own secreted sebum. You also know that sebum is imperative for the health and looks of your curls and that, without this precious oil, your mane will be headed towards dead rat camp. The question now arises, if shampoos are such powerful cleaning agents, how frequently should I use them then? Well, the answer is a bit more complicated than giving you a fixed number since shampooing frequency is quite individual and requires some trial and error to find out.

It is imperative for you to find out your optimal shampooing frequency so as to sport an awesome mane because an optimal shampooing frequency strives for sebum harmony: you don't remove sebum too frequently, nor do you encourage too much of its accumulation. Moreover, it is not only excess sebum that needs to be removed but also any hairstyling products (e.g. hair gel) that you may use and that too need to be removed. Thus, the need for your hair to be cleaned daily calls for you to strive to find out your specific and optimal shampooing frequency with the knowledge and guidelines that are to follow. Don't worry, I won't have you doing potentially-embarrassing kitchen experiments like I have been doing during all these years; finding out one's optimal shampooing frequency is actually a smooth and drama-free experience.

Before we dig into the whole finding out of your optimal shampooing frequency, I'd like to first put a full stop here and quickly tell you in the next 2 paragraphs about something that may very well go against what you thought was correct shampooing wisdom. An awesome mane requires you to keep an open mind and have a freshly-reset brain, so it is very important to make sure that you understand what you will read now.

Not shampooing your hair daily is neither wrong nor unhygienic. Your mane will not become a dirty, foul, stinking, awful-looking beast; on the contrary, it will look, smell and feel better. My personal experience and my experience advising other men in hair-grooming matters have proven that shampooing daily is not the optimal way to go about having a great mane of curls. Bear in mind that we are not talking here about walking around with a dead rat bouncing on top of your head or even having average-looking curls; we are talking about and aiming for kicking your curly mane up a few extra notches to mane awesomeness. Even curly haired women don't shampoo every day, and while we men can get away with rocking the caveman look if need be, 99% of women don't fancy rocking awful and smelly hair, hence there's certainly a merit to not shampooing daily if you have curly hair.

Back in the '60s and with the advent of the hippie movement, shampoos were cunningly marketed by the big hair care companies as bottled solutions for having clean and pure hair, or, in other words, you would not be a hippie if you shampooed your hair. Essentially, the more you shampooed, the less of a hippie you were, and thus housewives would rush daily to the bathroom to wash any hippiness off their children and keep it away as if it were some sort of demonic force. The myth prevailed as it was successfully ingrained in consumers' minds, and shampooing daily is still seen as the proper and only method to keeping one's hair clean. In a, perhaps, demonic paradox too, the vast majority of curly haired men who have come to me sporting a dead rat and seeking hair advice had the same hair-grooming flaw in common: they all shampooed their curly mane daily. Cutting their shampooing frequency to lower than daily was the easiest and most convenient way to quickly fix their curls; needless to say, not shampooing daily does work and is far from demonic!

So, after the above interesting paragraphs refuting conventional shampooing dogma, the question still remains, what is the optimal shampooing frequency to use? The answer is, it depends!

The optimal shampooing frequency to use is highly individual and will vary from one male to another although just about all curly men benefit from shampooing anywhere from "every other day" to "once a week", and it is within this range that you have to find out your optimal frequency. Such disparity in frequency among males is because we all have different scalps, curly hair types, hair lengths, preferences and lives. These are the main factors influencing the optimal shampooing frequency in men:

- Sebum secretion: this is defined by your genetic makeup, and some men just secrete more sebum than others.

- Hair products: some types of hair products tend to leave quite a bit of residue on the hair strands and scalp, which means that shampooing frequency has to be a bit higher than if you weren't using these products. Waxes and pomades are among the heaviest residue-leaving hair products.

- Exposure to the environment: if you move around environments that encourage nasty stuff to stick to your hair (e.g. bars where people smoke, or you spend a lot of time outdoors), you should then schedule a shampooing session after each given exposure.

- Curly hair type: the tighter the curl type, the better it will fare with a lower shampooing frequency as these curl types have the highest predisposition to dryness and not being fully sebuminised.

- Hair length: the longer your hair, the lower your shampooing frequency should be when compared to short hair.

- Preference: at the end of the day, if you prefer one frequency over the rest, your chances of adhering to it over the long term are higher.

In terms of the benefits that you will be obtaining from finding out your optimal shampooing frequency, they are:

- Hair will be less frizzy and dry.

- Shinier and more vigorous-looking hair.

- Less propensity for your curls to tangle.

- Potentially-less scalp irritation from the harsh ingredients of shampoo (for those with sensitive skin).

- More convenience as you don't have to go through the whole shampooing ordeal every day (you will be cutting down time from your hair grooming routine).

- Less of the unknown stuff that can be potentially absorbed by the scalp.

In other words, by finding out your optimal shampooing frequency, you will be obtaining the many bonuses that will pave the way for an awesome mane.

Now, on to the good stuff.

To find out what optimal shampooing frequency is best for you, you must ease off the shampooing slowly. If you shampoo daily, your scalp is literally hooked on the stuff so just stopping the shampoo altogether is going to make you go through some harsh shampoo withdrawals, which I can attest to being composed of your hair looking and feeling very greasy, with your scalp itching 24/7. You must drop your shampooing frequency slowly; take your time as, after all, your mane relationship is lifelong, so there is no need to rush its knowing.

For starters, I want you to start skipping the shampooing every other day, or what I call 1 on/1 off, with "on" being your shampooing day and "off" being your non-shampooing day. Thus, with 1 on/1 off, you shampoo one day, skip the shampoo the following day, and then you shampoo again on the third day. This is your starting point.

From there onwards, you will start adding an extra "off" day every 2 weeks until you find out your optimal shampooing frequency. However, in order to know when you have hit jackpot with your optimal frequency as you keep adding "off" days every 2 weeks, you should be striving to satisfy the following 5 indicators to shampooing frequency, which you will be reviewing at the end of each 2-week cycle per added "off" day. It will be once you satisfy these 5 indicators that you will have found out your optimal shampooing frequency:

1) <u>Your hair looks fuller:</u> you will notice that your hair will mysteriously start to look fuller and with more volume. This is completely normal and is a desired effect as your hair is starting to get optimal sebum coating and you are achieving sebum harmony.

2) <u>Your hair will start to look less dry:</u> again, sebum will now be allowed to optimally coat the hair strands, which means that your hair will look less dry.

3) <u>Your hair will feel smoother upon running your fingers through it:</u> dry hair feels hay-like whereas greasy hair feels hard to the touch (disgusting, even). Optimally-shampooed hair, on the other hand, feels smooth and light upon touching and feeling it, even when no hair products have been applied priorly.

4) <u>Your scalp doesn't have an overaccumulation of sebum:</u> an excess of sebum will manifest itself as small wax-like particles, which you will be able to notice in the mirror at first glance. You will know that you have lowered your shampooing

frequency too much as these tiny particles are the first to show up when you are not shampooing with enough frequency.

5) <u>Your curls look defined:</u> as you approach your optimal shampooing frequency, you will notice that your curls will become more defined. Instead of looking like tumbleweed (dry hair) or looking plastered (greasy hair), your curls will look more shapely, and you will be able to see the enhanced curl definition in the mirror and so will others.

The above 5 indicators are somewhat subjective. What is fuller to you, may not be as full to me, but the point remains; you will be noticing an increasing cosmetic benefit on your curls as they start to look fuller, less dry, smoother, more defined, and no particles of overaccumulated sebum are to be seen on your mane. However, when in doubt, ask yourself, would I let my hair look like this if I were to go on a first date with a hot chick? That cue will tell you in an instant if you have currently hit your optimal shampooing frequency (married guys: instead, ask your ladies what they think of the gradual change in your curls, I don't want to incite you folks to think of any women other than your "one and only"!).

All right, so now that you know the above 5 indicators and what to look for when striving to find out your optimal shampooing frequency, this is how you will actually go about it:

- Hold the aforementioned initial 1 on/1 off shampooing frequency for 2 weeks. This is your starting frequency.

- Assess after those 2 weeks, and try to do the actual assessment when your hair has been fully dried and has no hairstyling products applied. Is your hair looking better? Have you satisfied the 5 indicators? If yes, you have found out your optimal frequency. If not, add another "off" day so that now you will be doing 1 on/2 off for the next 2 weeks. If you have found quite profound benefits with 1 on/1 off, you can still try 1 on/2 off if you fancy seeing whether you can get further cosmetic benefits or not.

- Reassess at the end of the 2 weeks with 1 on/2 off. Satisfied the 5 indicators? If yes, 1 on/2 off is for you. If not, add another "off" day for a 1 on/3 off schedule to be implemented for the next 2 weeks.

- After those 2 weeks of 1 on/3 off, reassess again and compare your results with the ideal results strived for in the 5 indicators. If you have satisfied them, then 1 on/3 off is your optimal frequency. If there is still some more room for improvement, add another "off" day for a new schedule of 1 on/4 off to be implemented for the next 2 weeks.

- And so on and so forth.

See the approach? You will continue to add an extra "off" day to your shampooing frequency until you satisfy the 5 indicators. Play it by the ear and don't make it complicated, you will already see results from 1 on/1 off, and from there onwards it is a matter of reassessing after each 2-week cycle per extra "off" day added. If you find out that after the given 2 weeks of your newly-tried frequency, the 5 factors have regressed instead of continued to progress, then go back to your previous shampooing frequency as the one causing you to regress is not the optimal one at that time.

Do not panic if it takes you many weeks and you end up with a 1 on/7 off shampooing frequency or an even lower frequency of shampoo use; this is all completely normal, and your shampooing frequency will vary according to your unique set of circumstances as I explained earlier in this sub-subsection. Likewise, your shampooing frequency may have to be adjusted at times according to changes in your lifestyle. If you start going out more to bars where people smoke, or if you grow your hair longer (to give you 2 examples), you may need to alter your frequency. You should see your shampooing frequency as a readjustable process, which you will have to fine-tune as your hair-related circumstances change. Use the satisfying of the 5 indicators as your gauge to whether your current shampooing frequency is working or if you need to tweak it.

Since you will be experimenting with your shampooing frequency, it is imperative that you leave the rest of your hair grooming routine intact during the timespan that it takes you to find out your optimal shampooing frequency. You will read later about the recommended hair grooming routine to use, but, essentially, the routine that you will be using during this timespan is based on having a fixed set of secondary actions for your shampooing days and a fixed set of secondary actions for your non-shampooing days. Ergo, due to your shampooing frequency being central to your hair grooming routine, it is best that you stick to a generic hair grooming routine while you find out your optimal shampooing frequency for the first time.

Your optimal shampooing frequency is not static, and once you have found it out, you can modify it in the future whenever you notice that the 5 indicators are starting to take a hit due to external factors. Having said that, you now have the template and knowledge to find out (initially) and modify (later) your shampooing frequency as needed so that you are always using an optimal frequency, this being in itself a key element in achieving and maintaining your awesome mane.

The Sebum Coating method

Just because you will not be shampooing on some days, it doesn't mean that you should stop cleaning your hair altogether! On your non-shampooing days (i.e. "off" days), you will still go about your hair grooming routine, soaking your hair with running water and then cleaning, conditioning and styling your mane. It will be on these "off" days that you will be doing the Sebum Coating method; do not be put off by the name because, just like with the optimal shampooing method, the Sebum Coating method is a convenient and fast method to getting your curls looking the part.

The Sebum Coating method consists of using your fingers to spread the scalp sebum across the whole length of the hair strands (i.e. sebuminise) so as to manually aid your curls in getting coated with this precious endogenous oil. This sebuminising method is performed on the days that you do not shampoo as these are the days when your secreted sebum is not removed by the shampoo. Moreover, the Sebum Coating method acts as a mild hair cleaner, removing any accumulated dust or mild residue from hair products as your fingers manually remove dirt through mechanical friction. Thus, the action of the Sebum Coating method is two-fold: to condition the hair by spreading the scalp sebum and to clean the hair via mechanical friction from the manual spreading motion. By doing the Sebum Coating method, you will be be keeping your hair conditioned and dirt free on your "off" days.

To do the Sebum Coating method, you need to completely soak your hair in water as if you were going to shampoo and then run your fingers gently through several hair locks at a time, with the finger-running motion starting from the base of the grabbed locks (scalp) and running to the very end of their length (tip). You run your fingers through the set of grabbed locks as water runs on it, and you only run your fingers through each set of locks once. The most efficient way to run your fingers is to pinch the thumb, index and middle fingers against the base of the locks and then move the fingers smoothly through the locks' length all the way to the tip.

Remember those 6 scalp segments that you will be using to apply the shampoo on your shampooing days (forehead, centre, both sides, vertex and nape)? Use the same pairing of segments, and simultaneously grab sets of hair locks from each segment at a time. Aim to grab as much hair as you can in about 1-inch-wide sets; typically, you will grab 3 to 10 hair locks in each 1-inch-wide set (depending on how thick your locks are naturally), and you can use wider sets or go lock by lock if you want to spend more time doing the Sebum Coating method (remember, a lock is nothing more than a group of hair strands growing next to each other and in the same direction). Just run your fingers once through each set of grouped locks, and then move on to the next set. Make sure that water is running on the set of hair locks that you are working on as you run your fingers, with the water being of a lukewarm temperature (not too hot, not too cold). Run your fingers fast and smoothly, avoiding any pulling of the locks; you are merely trying to spread a thin film of oil from the base of the locks to their tips, so there is no hair pulling involved here.

The point of the Sebum Coating method is to not only clean the hair but to also mobilise and spread the secreted scalp sebum with the help of your fingers so that the sebum can then coat the whole length of the hair strands. Since sebum is secreted by the sebaceous glands continuously and due to the tendency of sebum to stay close to the scalp in curly hair, this oily substance needs your help so as to travel across the entire length of the hair strands. Get your fingers working with the explained motion; you will even sometimes feel the sebum in your fingertips as you do the Sebum Coating method. Sebum is somewhat greasy yet odourless and clear, unless it has accumulated excessively as then it will resemble wax, and it will mean that you still haven't achieved your optimal shampooing frequency.

Overall, the Sebum Coating method will take you a maximum of 2 minutes to implement on all of your hair, less time once you master it. Remember, you only run your fingers once per set of hair locks, and you do it smoothly and fast; if the Sebum Coating method is taking you more than 2 minutes to complete, then aim to grab wider sets of locks. You can do the Sebum Coating method as frequently as you want although, as a bare minimum, you must implement it on your non-shampooing days for your first cleaning stage. If you are still unsure about what constitutes a lock of hair and how it relates to the Sebum Coating method, refer to Question 10 in Chapter 8 "Questions & Answers: Because They Will Come".

Since the Sebum Coating method acts as a cleaning and conditioning agent, on your non-shampooing days the Sebum Coating method can also be used to substitute a conditioner for the second stage (conditioning) of your hair grooming routine. What's more is that the actual action of the Sebum Coating method in the first stage as a hair cleaner already conditions the hair as the fingers spread the sebum, so there's no need to repeat the Sebum Coating method a second time for the conditioning stage. In other words, on your non-shampooing days, you can fuse both the first and second stages of your hair grooming routine by just performing the Sebum Coating method and then moving on to the third styling stage.

The Sebum Coating method can also be performed on shampooing days if you so prefer. In this instance, the Sebum Coating method would be done prior to shampooing, meaning that the Sebum Coating method would the first secondary action of your hair grooming routine on the given shampooing day. The biggest benefit of doing the Sebum Coating method before shampooing is that you will enhance the hair-cleaning action of the shampoo as you will have spread any excess sebum close to the scalp with your fingers before cleaning the scalp with the shampoo. It is up to you if you want to do the Sebum Coating method on your shampooing days, but you certainly need to do the Sebum Coating method on your non-shampooing days for your first cleaning stage.

The Sebum Coating method is extremely useful, so do not skip it! With this method, you will encourage the optimal sebum coating of your curls while cleaning the hair, and you will be noticing your hair looking smoother, shinier and more defined once you get good at it.

A shampooing note on curl types and hair length

As you can see in the table that follows (Figure 19), shampooing frequency typically differs according to curl type and hair length although the frequencies below are just guidelines, and you may require a specific shampooing frequency that differs from what is typical for your curl type and given hair length.

Figure 19 – Typical shampooing frequency per curl type and hair length category (High= 1 on/1 off, Very low= 1 on/7 off)

	CURLY HAIR TYPES				
	Type I	Type II	Type III	Type IV	Type V
Near-shaved	High	High	Moderate	Moderate	Moderate
Short	High	Moderate	Moderate	Low	Low
Medium	Moderate	Moderate	Low	Low	Very low
Long	Moderate	Low	Low	Very low	Very low

As a rule of thumb, the tighter your curl type is, the lower the shampooing frequency that you will use because coils and kinks (Type III, IV and V) have a bigger issue than waves (Type I and II) in getting coated optimally with sebum. Likewise, the tighter the curl type, the higher the predisposition to dryness, which means that shampoo should be used infrequently and the Sebum Coating method should be emphasised on every non-shampooing day to ensure the daily cleaning of one's curls while providing extra conditioning to the hair strands with the spread sebum.

When it comes to hair length, for every incremental length category that you grow your hair to (e.g. from short to medium), you should reduce your shampooing frequency by adding 1 extra "off" day, whatever your already established shampooing frequency may be. And the reverse goes for cutting your hair and going down in length category (e.g. from medium to short): you will increase your shampooing frequency by removing 1 "off" day per length category gone down to.

For example, say you followed the method to working out your optimal shampooing frequency for your 0.5-inch curls (short-length category), and it turns out that a 1 on/2 off is the optimal frequency for you at that hair length. You then decide to grow your curls to 3 inches (medium length), and continue with your 1 on/2 off shampooing frequency right until your hair reaches the medium-length category (2-inch mark); you would then automatically add 1 extra "off" day to your current shampooing frequency, hence decreasing your shampooing frequency to 1 on/3 off as your curls have grown past the 2-inch mark. If, after some months, you decide to cut your hair and go from a medium length to a short length, then you would automatically remove 1 "off" day from your then-current 1 on/3 off to have a new shampooing frequency of 1 on/2 off as your hair has been cut to a short length (i.e. gone down 1 length category).

The reason behind decreasing your shampooing frequency as your hair grows is because the longer your hair is, the harder it is for your curls to get coated with sebum. Once your hair grows to a medium length and beyond, you need to pay special attention to how your hair is coated with sebum as optimal sebum coating is key to maintaining a great-looking mane. You must really get good at the Sebum Coating method and think of cleaning your hair as the first stage in your hair grooming routine that is made of 3 equally important elements: shampooing method, shampooing frequency and the Sebum Coating method.

Of course, the above rules of thumbs are just that, rules of thumb; they are there to serve you as guidelines to fast-tracking the finding out of your specific shampooing frequency, the latter being an element of your hair grooming routine that will not only vary according to your curl type and your hair length but that will also vary according to the unique set of circumstances that you find yourself in during different periods of your lifetime.

A shampooing note on when your hair has too much residue

Over time, too much residue from hairstyling products may accumulate in your hair and both shampooing and the Sebum Coating method won't be enough to remove the residue fully. This typically occurs in cases where you have been using hairstyling products erroneously for too long. As you will learn in the section of this chapter that is dedicated to the styling stage of your hair grooming, you must apply your hairstyling products in a particular smart manner; otherwise, you run the risk of having layers of unremoved hairstyling products coating your hair shafts and drying the hair from the inside as no moisture from external sources is allowed into the shafts. The excess of unremoved hairstyling-product residue creates a noticeable effect by which your hair will feel heavy, greasy, hay-like and will loose its natural defined shape.

Through the No Shampoo method and your hair-grooming routine, you will be routinely cleaning the hair with great efficiency and effectiveness. However, you are not always guaranteed to be cleaning your hair optimally or to be applying the hairstyling products correctly, especially as you begin your journey to great-looking and convenient hair, and unremoved hairstyling products may start to pile up in your hair. Thus, it is in such scenarios where residue in your hair is not being responsive to your hair grooming that you must insert a special type of shampoo: a clarifying shampoo. This type of shampoo is quite similar to conventional shampoos except clarifying shampoos offer a stronger hair-cleaning functionality, meaning they are powerful shampoos and should not be used often (i.e. with a lesser frequency than your conventional shampoo).

Once you're coasting along with your newly-found optimal shampooing frequency, you may, at times, find your hair coated in an excess of residue caused by specific hair-grooming mistakes you've done as you're still new to the workings of the hair-equation system (e.g. a common mistake is using too much hairstyling product every day for weeks at a time); it is thus in these scenarios that you can use a clarifying shampoo to remove this unwanted accumulation of residue. Likewise, you can use a clarifying shampoo right at the end of the period covering the finding out of your optimal shampooing frequency; once you have found out such essential frequency of shampoo use, then use a clarifying shampoo and start afresh with an uber-cleaned scalp and locks.

Contrary to the shampoo application for the No Shampoo method, the clarifying shampoo should be allowed on all of your hair's length, not just on the scalp and segment of the hair strands closest to the scalp, for the goal is to remove absolutely everything that is coating your hair (whether good or bad) regardless of location. When you find your hair coated in a permanent layer of hairstyling products that is unresponsive to your usual shampooing and Sebum Coating method, then schedule a clarifying shampoo session as soon as possible and treat the session as that of a shampooing day (i.e. follow with a normal conditioner and styling product). Resume your normal shampooing frequency after the clarifying-shampoo session.

Second stage – Conditioning

Conditioning is the second stage of your hair grooming routine, and it is performed after you have rinsed the shampoo or implemented the Sebum Coating method. Your conditioning action is performed with a conditioner: a hair grooming product that does its conditioning job by allowing the hair strands to retain moisture (i.e. prevents dryness) while providing gloss. Moreover, conditioners enhance the slip between curls and, overall, improve the manageability of one's mane. Thus, conditioners are great weapons for you to have in your hair grooming arsenal because dryness is a big issue that wreaks havoc in our curly manes, and conditioners tackle this issue from the very root (no pun intended).

Your scalp already secretes an awesome conditioner: your own sebum. Unfortunately, sebum can't always do its job properly, and artificial conditioners provide an extra aid to your mane to make your locks look great. Now that you know how to make the most of your own natural conditioner via the Sebum Coating method, it is time to know how to use conditioners as these products will provide an extra advantage, on top of your own sebum, to make your mane awesome.

There are 2 types of conditioners that are of need to you: normal conditioners and leave-in conditioners. Normal conditioners need to be applied and left on your hair for 2 minutes after having cleaned the hair, and they are rinsed after the 2-minute count. On the other hand, leave-in conditioners are used when styling your mane in the third stage and are not rinsed or washed away until you clean your hair again. Incidentally, normal conditioners are used in the second stage of your hair grooming, and leave-in conditioners are used in the third stage within the same routine (i.e. leave-ins are used in the styling stage, not in the conditioning stage). However, both types of conditioners have the same main action: to condition the hair strands, and they can be used concomitantly on the same day.

Both types of conditioners are key in building your awesome mane, and you will benefit from them extensively if you use them the correct way. Conditioners are of special use to men with the higher-end curls (III to V) because these curl types have the biggest issue with dryness and in getting coated with sebum, and because tangling of the hair strands is a very prominent issue the tighter one's curls are. However, both types of conditioners are of great use to all curl types, and you should have them in your hair grooming arsenal for an awesome mane regardless of your curl type.

Normal conditioners

Normal conditioners are predominantly used on your shampooing days following the rinsing of the shampoo, although they can also be used on your non-shampooing days after the Sebum Coating method. Regarding their name, normal conditioners are simply labelled as "conditioners" by hair care companies, but I prefer to call them "normal conditioners" in this book so as to avoid confusion with leave-in conditioners.

Normal conditioners are hair products that leave a thin film coating the hair strands in a similar way as to how sebum is intended to do. The thin film left by normal conditioners acts to seal in moisture into the hair strands while smoothing out the cuticle of the hair shaft, which translates into a cosmetic benefit to your mane. Normal conditioners also have a lubricating effect, meaning that they are great tools to keep your locks free of tangles. Lastly, normal conditioners provide gloss (i.e. make the hair shinier) and ultimately allow you to manage your curls with more ease.

You should use a normal conditioner straight after you rinse the shampoo from your hair. Pour the conditioner on your palms and rub them together so as to spread the conditioner on the fingers of both your hands, leaving a thick film of conditioner coating the fingers. Then, use your fingers to apply the conditioner to all of your hair, aiming to coat the hair strands with a film of conditioner from mid-length to the tips. What you have just read is very important: do not apply the conditioner to the segment of the hair strands close to the scalp or on the scalp itself (i.e. the reverse of the shampoo application).

As men with curly hair, our main mane problem lies in the area between the mid-length and the tip of the hair shaft as this is the segment of the hair that is predisposed to dryness. While the Sebum Coating method will maximise the spread of sebum across the length of the hair strands, it is only normal that a good chunk of the sebum will remain closest to where it is secreted from: the scalp. Thus, you must emphasise the application of the conditioner from mid-length all the way up to the tip of the hair for that's where the conditioner is most needed.

Use plenty of normal conditioner and generously, but be careful if you have short-length hair as it is easy to get the conditioner on your scalp unintentionally. After applying it to your hair, leave the conditioner on without rinsing for 2 minutes while you continue grooming and cleaning the rest of your body in the shower. Once the 2 minutes are over, rinse the conditioner with running water, making sure that the washed-away conditioner doesn't go in your eyes because, just like with shampoo, you don't want the stuff near your eyes. About 30 seconds is more than enough to wash away all the conditioner from your hair.

Again, normal conditioners are used in the second stage of your shampooing days and following the rinsing of the shampoo. However, you can also use normal conditioners on the days that you do not shampoo (i.e. non-shampooing days) but only after the Sebum Coating method, not before. Essentially, your own secreted sebum is your de facto conditioner on your non-shampooing days, yet you can also add extra conditioning on these "off" days by using a normal conditioner after the Sebum Coating method.

Indeed, while the Sebum Coating method is more than enough for your conditioning action on your non-shampooing days, occasionally using normal conditioners on your "off" days can be beneficial especially for those men with curls in the higher curl type range (Type IV-V) as well as for those men with long hair. The good thing is that using a very high frequency of normal conditioner use (e.g. daily) will not have much of a negative impact on your mane as opposed to using a too-high shampooing frequency (e.g. daily), so feel free to introduce normal conditioners on your "off" days if you are keen to experiment. A good starting point that I have used in the past is to introduce normal conditioners on 50% of my non-shampooing days, but you can play around with higher percentages without fearing a dead rat. In any case, do remember that normal conditioners must be used on your shampooing days, and any further use on your "off" days will be subject to trial and error as well as personal preference.

Leave-in conditioners

Leave-in conditioners work as normal conditioners and have the same purpose. The difference is that leave-ins are left on the hair and can also be used to style one's hair as a hairstyling product. Unlike the normal variety, you don't apply the leave-in conditioner in the shower, and you don't rinse it either. You get out of the shower; you dry your hair so that it is left in a damp state, and you then apply the leave-in conditioner to your curls as you work your chosen hairstyle. Consequently, leave-ins are used in the third styling stage and not in the second conditioning stage despite leave-ins having a main conditioning action like normal conditioners have.

To use a leave-in conditioner, the same application rule goes as with normal conditioners: do not get the leave-in anywhere near the scalp, only apply from mid-length to the tip of the hair. Put some in your fingers and work your way through your curls to coat the hair with a film of leave-in conditioner, then proceeding to style your mane. Some leave-in conditioners also come in handy sprays; yet, no matter what their packaging form is, the main action of a leave-in conditioner is to condition the hair, and all leave-ins are not to be rinsed and can be used as products to style the hair.

Leave-in conditioners should ideally be used for your styling stage on your non-shampooing days after the Sebum Coating method, although they can also be used daily and without regard to your shampooing frequency. They are of special value once your hair has reached a medium length, and leave-ins can be used in conjunction with other hairstyling products (leave-in conditioner first, then the other product) or used alone to style the hair. And as with normal conditioners, don't get the stuff on the scalp or in your eyes!

Conditioners, the Sebum Coating method and putting it all together

Normal and leave-in conditioners are great, but the Sebum Coating method is just as great. The 3 used together, however, works like magic.

The Sebum Coating method has an important hair-conditioning action apart from its also important hair-cleaning action, hence the Sebum Coating method satisfies the second conditioning stage of your hair grooming routine. The Sebum Coating method fuses both first and second stages on your non-shampooing days, and it allows you to go straight to the third stage (i.e. styling) without having to use a normal conditioner as you'd otherwise do after your first stage on your shampooing days.

Normal conditioners are a must on your shampooing days. On your non-shampooing days, you can strictly soak your hair in water, do the Sebum Coating method and then get out of the shower to style your mane, skipping the normal conditioner. However, on your shampooing days, you must use a normal conditioner after rinsing the shampoo; once you have applied and rinsed the normal conditioner, you can then move on to the third styling stage.

In addition to the above, you can also include a normal conditioner for your second stage on your non-shampooing days after the Sebum Coating method: a good starting point is to use a normal conditioner on 50% of your non-shampooing days. Some men with the kinkiest of curls (Type V) may find out that they need to practically use normal conditioners every day without consideration to shampooing frequency and despite using the Sebum Coating method on their stipulated non-shampooing days.

Leave-in conditioners are very handy tools, and they can be used together with other hairstyling products (e.g. hair gel) to put your hair into a hairstyle. Leave-ins not only serve a conditioning purpose but they are also great hairstyling agents for those hairstyles in which hair doesn't need to be fixed into a position. Leave-in conditioners can be used every day, and they are very easy to remove the next time that you clean your hair with a shampoo or the Sebum Coating method. Ergo, when you are really pressed for time on your non-shampooing days, you can jump in the shower, do the Sebum Coating method, then move to styling your awesome mane with a leave-in conditioner and rush out the door with a moisturised and sebum-optimised head of curls.

As a drastic measure, you can even skip using a leave-in conditioner on your non-shampooing days, but, ideally and so as to ensure the conditioning of your mane, you should use a leave-in conditioner on your non-shampooing days as part of the third styling stage and after the Sebum Coating method. Once your hair reaches a medium length though, you will tangibly discover that using a leave-in conditioner on just about every day is the best way to keep your curls looking great. As a matter of fact, you may find that only using a leave-in conditioner as your de facto hairstyling product is the best way forward with your awesome mane.

For what is worth, many men who come to me for hair advice are not only unaware of what hair conditioners actually are, but they also have a wrong perception or attitude towards these hair grooming products. No, conditioners are not for girls; and, no, they will not require half of your morning to apply and use. As you have learnt in this section, both normal and leave-in conditioners are fundamental pieces of the conditioning action, and they are convenient and useful tools that will allow you to build your optimal hair grooming routine so as to sport an awesome mane.

Third stage – Styling

Styling your awesome mane is the third stage and final main action of your hair grooming routine, and it involves the following secondary actions:

1) Using the right hairstyling agent (i.e. hairstyling product) to get your mane looking as you want it to look. A leave-in conditioner is included here as one of the hairstyling agents available to use.

2) Knowing what you want as a hairstyle, and putting your mane into one.

3) Taking your hair from wet to damp (i.e. dry your hair) so as to prepare your curls for styling.

While I will cover a wide array of hairstyles available to you in the fifth chapter "Achieving The Physical Part: Putting Your Mane Together", it is best that this styling section is dedicated to outlining the different hairstyling agents available to you as well as the essentials of styling your awesome mane; it is only once you know these that you can truly make the most of any hairstyles you may so choose. You will read about the hairstyles recommended for each curl type in the fifth chapter so as to not have you overloaded with information in this chapter; thus, for now, let's us concentrate on the core of your styling stage.

Styling your mane is the last stage of the hair grooming process, and it is here where you can be a bit more casual and lax: curly hair that is properly moisturised will already look great without the need to style it. So long as you use shampoos smartly, make the most of your own sebum and use conditioners appropriately, you will already have the grooming foundation for your awesome mane. The styling puts the icing on the cake.

Hairstyling agents

Unfortunately, many men make the mistake of looking at hairstyling agents (i.e. hairstyling products) as the fix to their hair dramas without even considering that the solution to their dead rats may rest elsewhere. While our fellow straight haired men may get away with ignoring the preceding 2 stages of the hair grooming process and may actually find some benefit in merely searching for that "magic" hairstyling agent, we curly men cannot afford this privilege, and we must have the first 2 hair grooming stages optimised before proceeding with any hairstyling agents for the styling of our awesome manes.

Now that I have said the above and emphasised the importance of the 2 previous hair grooming stages, let's talk "awesome mane styling".

When it comes to styling curly hair, you can go solo (i.e. no hairstyling agent), or you can use a hairstyling agent or a blend of several. Hairstyling "agents" only differ from hairstyling "products" in that agents include not only all hairstyling commercial products but also include natural oils and butters, the latter 2 not necessarily sold as hair products and which can be found in food stores. Thus, I prefer to use "agents" as a term to denote any product, commercial or not, that can be used to style hair.

Overall, there are 8 main hairstyling agents that you can use for your mane:

1) Gel

2) Pomade

3) Wax

4) Mousse

5) Leave-in conditioner

6) Styling cream

7) Hair spray

8) Natural oils and butters

All of the above hairstyling agents differ in ingredients and functionality. What's more is that some are better suited to certain curl types. For example, men with curls Type I, II and III tend to benefit from hair gels and waxes, whereas those with Type IV and V curls tend to find leave-in conditioners, oils or going solo with an emphasis on the Sebum Coating method to be of greater benefit. You can find in Appendix XXIII, Appendix XXIV and Appendix XXV a series of tables listing the most suitable hairstyling agents per each curl type and hair length. Don't worry about these tables for now though, they will be most useful once you have understood and grasped the knowledge of this whole chapter, so leave their studying for later.

With hairstyling agents, you will find that you will need to experiment a little to find out the one (or a blend of) that is best suited to you. While in this section you will learn the details and guidelines to each hairstyling agent and how useful each is to a specific curl type, trialling different hairstyling agents (and even brands within each agent) will be of benefit to you especially since, at the end of the day, personal preference is key in choosing and adhering to one's hair grooming routine.

All of the 8 hairstyling agents are applied when you hair is damp, not wet or dry. That means that styling your mane as part of your hair grooming routine normally occurs in the morning when you are done in the shower and then get out of the shower to take your hair from wet to damp (i.e. dry your hair). Never style your mane when it has fully dried and isn't damp, only those with straight hair can pull this shortcut; either style your hair after you shower and the hair is damp, or quickly dampen your locks with water before applying your chosen hairstyling agent. Likewise, all these hairstyling agents are applied to your hair as you'd do with conditioners: from the hair strands' mid-length all the way to the tips, never close to the scalp (remember, shampoo is the only hair grooming product that you use on your scalp).

Because you, as a modern curly male, need to know what weapons you can have in your hair grooming arsenal for mane awesomeness, I will now go through each hairstyling agent available as well as their pros and cons so that you can decide for yourself which to use and integrate into the third stage of what constitutes your hair grooming routine. Do note, however, that hair care companies sometimes innovate the formulation of one of their hairstyling agents, having the agent behave differently than what would otherwise be expected; so, in terms of expectations, always treat any new hairstyling agent that you buy with caution.

Hair gel

Quite likely, you will already be familiar with hair gels. They come in a variety of "holds" (i.e. strengths), and they are great for Type I to IV curls ranging from short to medium length as hair gel is very useful to hold (secure in place) the hair in many hairstyles. Hair gel should be avoided by those men with Type V curls although "light hold" hair gel can be used in small quantities to provide the finishing touches for this tightest of curl types.

Pros:

- Lasts the whole day.

- Holds hair in place; awesome for hairstyles requiring hair to remain fixed.

- Great for sculpting a hairstyle (best for Type I-III curls, though).

- Wide variety of cool smells.

- Will define your curls.

Cons:

- Leaves residue on your hair.

- Tangles your curls, especially if they are Type V or long Type IV.

- Will impede your locks from fully hanging down.

- Strong hold gel can make long curls look like nasty crunchy sticks.

Hair pomade

Unlike hair gel, hair pomade doesn't dry fully, and it gives hair a shiny look. Hair pomade is best used on curls Type I to IV, ranging from short to medium length.

Pros:

- Lasts the whole day.

- Makes curls look slick.

- Makes hair shiny and glossy.

- Neutral smell.

- Will define curls.

- Will help hang down your curls.

Cons:

- Difficult to remove, leaves some residue.

- Can make hair look greasy if you apply too much (Types I and II, watch out for this one).

- Not the best hairstyling agent to hold hair in place.

Hair wax

Hair waxes are the more solid version of pomades. They are better than pomades for holding hair in place, and they do not dry fully either. Wax works best on short to medium-length Type I and II curls, and, unlike pomade, hair wax is a good option for hairstyles that encourage the defying of gravity.

- Lasts the whole day.

- Works good for holding hair in place.

- Great for sculpting a hairstyle (though hair gel is better).

- Gives a shiny look.

- Will define your curls.

Cons:

- Difficult to remove, leaves lots of residue.

- Will make Type IV and V curls look frizzy.

- Can leave hair looking greasy very fast, especially in Types I and II.

- Needs some more application time as you must pay extra attention to not get the hair wax on your scalp.

- Not suitable for long-length curls.

Hair mousse

Hair mousse is great for making your hair look more voluminous. It still holds the hair in place, but it also adds a volumising element to your styling. It is best used on Types I and II as these are the curl types that have the least natural volume of all curly hair types, so hair mousse is a great tool for hairstyles aiming to style the hair with a big-volume emphasis. Hair mousse works the greatest on medium to long-length curls and can be used with a hair dryer to enhance the acquired extra hair volume (apply the hair mousse first, then use the hair dryer).

Pros:

- Works reasonably well to hold hair in place.

- Will add plenty of volume to your hair, even if your curls are not Type I and II.

- Will define your curls.

- Works great for hairstyles requiring "puffing out" (volumising) and the use of a hair dryer.

- Easy to wash off.

- Will give a wet-look effect when combined with some hair spray.

- Unintentionally getting some on your scalp is not as bad as the rest of hairstyling agents.

Cons:

- Not great for sculpting hairstyles.

- Will not last the whole day if you are active (e.g. you spend time outdoors or in the gym).

- Will give the nasty "crunchy stick" look if you overdo it.

- Not the best hairstyling agent for short-length curls nor higher-end curls (IV-V).

Leave-in conditioner

Leave-in conditioners not only work as de facto normal conditioners but they also work as hairstyling agents to use if you want your curls to be hanging down and looking glossy. Leave-in conditioners are useful for all curl types and lengths, and they can be used alone as a hairstyling agent or together with other hairstyling agents. Leave-in conditioners are also a necessary item when your curls reach a medium length regardless of your curl type. If you want to use a leave-in with other hairstyling agents, always apply the leave-in first.

Pros:

- Conditions and moisturises your curls like no other hairstyling agent.

- Great to use if you want your hair to hang down (best done in combination with a styling cream).

- Easy to remove.

- Doesn't dry excessively like hair gel does.

- Overdoing it will not make your hair freak out like hair gel or hairspray will do.

- Works great in combination with any other hairstyling agents especially hair gel and styling creams.

- Convenient; you can apply it quickly and be done in seconds.

- Will help define your curls.

- Provides ample slip to the curls, which will help in keeping your mane tangle free.

- Unintentionally getting some on your scalp is not as bad as the rest of hairstyling agents.

Cons:

- Doesn't hold hair in place.

- Not good for sculpting a hairstyle.

- Not suitable for short-length curls as a standalone hairstyling agent, combine with another hairstyling agent for best cosmetic results if you have a short-length mane.

- Should be used daily when curls are at a medium or long length (though its application is fast and convenient).

Styling cream

A styling cream is a neater version of a pomade and is great for taming frizz and adding shine. Styling creams add weight to the hair, so they are very useful to weight down your curls if you want them to hang down at lengths in which your curly hair still defies gravity in a natural/no hair-product state. All curl types benefit from styling creams although this hairstyling agent is particularly suited for Type III to V curls at medium length and longer especially if used to make the curls hang down.

Pros:

- Great for defining your curls.

- Good at taming frizz and flyaway hairs.

- Adds shine with a wet-look effect.

- Adds weight to hair, which helps it to hang down at medium and long lengths.

Cons:

- Doesn't hold hair in place very well.

- Despite being lighter in residue than wax, it is still a nuisance to remove.

- Not optimal for short-length Type I and II curls (instead, use hair gel, pomade or wax).

- Can make hair look greasy if overdone.

Hair spray

Hair spray is used to harden your curls and hold them in place like no other. It can be used on any curl type, and it should be viewed as the finishing touch to secure your hair for those hairstyles or occasions in which you want to rock a certain look day long. When used with hair mousse, it can give a wet look too (apply the hair mousse first, then use the spray).

Pros:

- Great for securing hair in place.

- Will last the whole day.

- Won't make your hands stench with product residue.

Cons:

- Easy to overdo it and have your hair looking like it is made of cardboard.

- Difficult to remove as it needs plenty of water to soften back the hair.

- Not a good option for Type IV and V curls (instead, use hair gel to harden your curls).

- You really don't want to get the stuff in your eyes (or your face, for that matter).

- Potential to inhale stuff you could do best without inhaling.

Natural oils and butters

That's right, you can also use natural oils and butters to style your hair! Coconut oil, olive oil, shea butter and jojoba oil are great agents to style your hair with, and they also aid in keeping your locks moisturised. Natural oils and butters provide the best results to those manes that are at least a medium length and range from Type III to Type V curl types although all curl types can benefit from natural oils and butter. Always use a minimal amount (think pea size) and approach using natural oils and butters to style your hair with a "less is more" attitude. Oils and butters can be used on any day of your hair grooming schedule, and you can think of them as being natural complements to your own sebum. To use butters, simply melt your chosen one by rubbing your hands together (do not apply the butter in a solid state).

Pros:

- Will make your hair look slick and shiny.

- Will condition your hair as a natural complement to your sebum.

- Doesn't dry excessively.

- Will help in defining your curls.

- Will add weight and thus help to make your curls hang down.

- Is a natural alternative, so you are ensured to not be absorbing unknown added chemicals through your scalp.

Cons:

- Extremely easy to overdo it and have your hair looking greasy.

- Not good for holding hair in place.

- Moderately difficult to remove (if you overdo it though, it will be a nightmare to remove).

- Takes longer to apply than other hairstyling agents as you have to be careful to not get the oil or butter on your scalp (same extra caution as with hair wax).

- Start with very small amounts for Types I and II curls as it can make this curl type appear greasy very fast.

- Some natural oils and butters can give off a natural smell if you use too much (fancy walking around smelling like a coconut?).

- It can stain your shirt collars if you have medium or long-length curls and you use too much.

How to style your curls

Ditch your hair brush, ditch it now!

The above is one of the first things that I say to those curly men who come to me seeking hair advice. Hair brushes work great for straight hair, but, for curly hair, they are the enemy. Hair brushes will break the curl pattern of your hair, and they will make your hair frizzy in an instant; hardly what an awesome mane should look like. Pocket combs and conventional combs are just as bad and will cause you to be pulling your curls constantly, which will not only damage the hair shaft of your hair but also your hair follicles.

To style your mane, you must either use your fingers or use a wide-tooth comb. For most of the time, however, I recommend you to use your fingers solely and only rely on the wide-tooth comb for hairstyles in which you want your mane to be held in place (e.g. a swept or slicked hairstyle). Wide-tooth combs are also great for undoing hair tangles, so it is in your interest to own one; the best quality wide-tooth combs are made out of wood or metal, avoid buying cheap plastic ones as they will chip easily.

With regards to applying your chosen hairstyling agent, coat your fingers with the agent and then run your fingers through your damp hair as you put your hair into your chosen hairstyle, trying to get most of the hairstyling agent on the segment of the hair strands from mid-shaft to the tip (as you'd do with conditioners). Once the hairstyling agent is applied and your hair has been styled with your fingers, you can then use the wide-tooth comb to give the finishing touches and directions to your mane, or you can continue using your fingers for the finishing touches of the hairstyle.

I must emphasise again that you have to use your chosen hairstyling agent on damp hair as this is a point that many curly men forget. Hairstyling agents won't work optimally on fully-dried curly hair, so having your mane damp is they way to go for its optimal styling. Once the hairstyling agent has been applied successfully to your damp hair, you are ready to leave the door with an awesome mane while your hair air-dries on its own to a fully-dried state as you go about your day.

How to dry your hair after the shower

Part of the styling stage and a secondary action in itself, drying your hair is performed so as to take your hair from wet or soaked to damp. Typically, drying your hair occurs after you finish showering, and it is done prior to applying the hairstyling agents to your hair.

There are 2 options available to dry your hair: shaking your head or using a towel. The point of drying your hair is to remove the excess water from it so that you leave the hair damp; you should never dry your hair until it loses all the moisture gained from having wetted it in the first place.

The Shakeout is the colloquial name for shaking your head to remove the excess water and thus effectively dry your hair to a damp state without the use of a towel or cloth. As the name implies, you simply shake your head sideways and back and forth, allowing the water to drip from your hair. The Shakeout method is best used on medium and long-length hair since you need to have enough length to move the mass of hair as you shake your head. A spin-off of the Shakeout method is the Finger Shakeout: rapidly pass the fingers of both your hands over your hair, aiming to flick the water off the hair; the Finger Shakeout works best on short hair.

The second method is towel-drying, which is the preferred method for many males as it is more efficient than the Shakeout method in removing excess water. The main issue with towel-drying, however, is that it can cause tangling of your locks as well as frizz if not done right.

To optimally towel-dry, gently pass the towel over your mane as if you were literally caressing your scalp and hair, squeezing the curls with the towel in your hand to let the excess water drip. Do not vigorously rub the towel against your scalp because this will lead to the tangling of your mane and will make your hair frizz rapidly. It is very important that you gently pass the towel and squeeze the curls with the towel in your hand if you choose this hair-drying method. Moreover, I recommend you to use an old cotton T-shirt instead of a towel to dry your curls since most bath towels have a rough surface and cotton T-shirts are much smoother and easier on the curls (simply use cotton T-shirts that you no longer wear). Towel-drying is a great option for all hair lengths and curl types so long as you do it as recommended.

You can mix and match the hair-drying methods, but, whatever method you choose, the goal is to have your hair damp so as to be able to apply the hairstyling agent. After the hairstyling agent has been applied and the hair has been styled, you do not manipulate your hair further; the hair will slowly achieve a final look as it dries fully (i.e. air-dries) on its own over the course of a couple of hours. This is where the Damp vs. Dry (DvD) effect comes into play, and your hair will invariably look somewhat different once it has fully dried; it all depends on your curl type, hair length, chosen hairstyle, chosen hairstyling agent, and your unique coil factor.

A note on using hair dryers

You are probably aware of what a hair dryer is, if anything because any of the females in your life (sister, mother or girlfriend/wife) quite likely has one and uses it frequently. Hair dryers, also known as blow dryers, are tools used to further dry your hair rapidly when your hair is damp instead of having to wait the few hours that your curly locks may take to fully air-dry on their own. Hair dryers are also of use for enhancing the volume of your curls and putting your hair into elaborate hairstyles.

The main problem with hair dryers is that these artefacts rely on the blowing of hot air to work their fast-drying magic. Excessive heat, especially as given out by hair dryers, can damage your awesome mane over the long term particularly if your hair care is subpar. If you want to use a hair dryer to dry your hair or enhance a hairstyle, follow these points:

- Use the coldest temperature available in the settings.

- Clip a diffuser to the hair drier to allow for optimal dissipation of the air expelled.

- Coat your hair with a special heat-protecting hair product prior to using the hair dryer.

- Do not use the hair dryer on wet or soaked hair; always dry your hair to a damp state (via the Shakeout or towel-drying) prior to drying your hair with the hair dryer.

- Do not go all out with the hair dryer to completely dry your hair, leave some moisture (i.e. dampness) in the hair as otherwise your hair will end up resembling a dead rat!

I recommend you to leave hair dryers out of the daily hair grooming equation and instead use these tools for specific occasions (e.g. when you want to rock a certain hairstyle). Hair dryers will do more bad than good if used daily as such frequent use will irreversibly damage your hair. For your daily hair grooming, use any of the 2 aforementioned hair-drying methods (Shakeout and/or towel-drying), and allow your awesome mane to fully air-dry naturally as you go about your day.

The 9-Minute Perfect Mane routine

To approach the grooming of your curly hair, you must regard the process as a routine. This is because grooming your curls is inherently a daily sequence of main and secondary actions, and to become better at something, you need to practise it frequently and in an orderly fashion; there's no 2 ways about this. What's more is that your awesome mane will be managed via your hair grooming routine in a slightly different manner according to the day as you alter the secondary actions in the 3 hair grooming stages. Regardless, your hair grooming routine will be built upon the template of having the 3 stages and main actions of cleaning, conditioning and styling performed on a daily basis. If you need another quick visual reference, see the table on Figure 18 (in the beginning of the chapter) for the 3 stages and their secondary actions (it is also found as Appendix XIX in the Appendix).

Of course, throughout the years, I have perfected my own hair grooming routine. Because I like to be my own lab rat and because all the hair grooming advice out there for curly hair involves massive amounts of time investment, I decided to really work on a hair grooming routine for my curls that would be convenient and that would yield great cosmetic results. This hair grooming routine that I came up with and perfected is called the 9-Minute Perfect Mane routine, and it involves everything you have read in this hair grooming chapter, albeit put together in a convenient and methodical manner. The 9-Minute Perfect Mane routine acts as the initial template to use in your awesome mane journey since it comprises the 3 hair grooming stages and helps you to visualise the flow of secondary actions.

I have been able to use the 9-Minute Perfect Mane routine while living in different countries, working on my career, training for a sport and partying my derriere off, so, with this hair grooming routine, you have the 3 hair grooming stages assembled into a convenient and optimal order and flow, ultimately suiting the modern male who needs time efficiency slammed into his daily hair management. The 9-Minute Perfect Mane routine is ideally done in a bathroom setting as it integrates the whole hair grooming process and shampooing is best done in the shower.

Here is the 9-Minute Perfect Mane routine, step by step (TT means Time Taken):

1) Jump in the shower. For best results, water should be lukewarm. Singing is recommended to get into the routine. (TT: 10 seconds)

2) Soak those curls with running water. Hair must be soaked in its entirety. (TT: 30 seconds)

3) Grab the shampoo. Squeeze out a fingertip amount and place it on the centre of the top of your head. (TT: 10 seconds)

4) Repeat Step 3 on your other 5 scalp segments: both sides of head, front, vertex and the area 4 inches above the nape. (TT: 50 seconds)

5) Pair the segments of the scalp and massage each segment with each hand simultaneously. Spread the shampoo to a 4-inch radius as you massage in a circular motion. Each paired segment is massaged for a count of 20 seconds. (TT: 60 seconds)

6) Rinse the shampoo with your head tilted forward or backward. (TT: 30 seconds)

7) Possibly change the song you've been singing. Up to you, but do it immediately.

8) Grab the normal conditioncr and squeeze it out on your fingers so that they (fingers) are coated in a thick film of conditioner. (TT: 10 seconds)

9) Work your fingers through your curls from mid-length to the tip, coating the hair plentifully with conditioner. (TT: 60 seconds)

10) Now clean your body. Make sure that you take 2 minutes to clean your body, which is the time that the conditioner should be left on your hair without rinsing. (TT: 120 seconds)

11) Rinse the conditioner. (TT: 30 seconds)

12) Get out of the shower. You are now going to style that mane. Start singing a new song if you so desire. (TT: 20 seconds)

13) Dry your hair via the Shakeout method and/or with a towel or cotton T-shirt so that your mane is left damp. (TT: 30 seconds)

14) Grab your chosen hairstyling agent and put some on your fingers. (TT: 10 seconds)

15) Run your fingers through your locks and style your mane as desired. Make sure that you don't get any of the hairstyling agent on the scalp. (TT: 60 seconds)

16) Wink at yourself. You are looking great and are ready to take the day with that awesome mane of yours.

The 9-Minute Perfect Mane routine contains 16 fluid steps and takes 530 seconds or 10 seconds under 9 minutes, from the moment you are about to get in the shower to the moment your hair is set and ready to go. Oh, and that is only on the days that you use shampoo; on your non-shampooing days, your average 9-Minute Perfect Mane routine can take even less (see Appendix XXI for reference). The above 9-Minute Perfect Mane routine serves as your initial template to then start modifying the secondary hair grooming actions to fit the routine according to your awesome mane's needs and preferences as well as whether it is a shampooing or non-shampooing day.

The 9-Minute Perfect Mane routine has you, in less than 9 minutes, sporting your awesome mane so that you can then get on with the rest of your day. We are talking less than 9 minutes to have a head of curls that looks awesome, a mane that you will be proud to be leaving the house with. Even with my own bushy coils and kinks, I still manage it in less than 9 minutes.

If I can do it with this beast, you too can do it, and, as you master the 9-Minute Perfect Mane routine, you will be able to gradually trim your routine's time to mere minutes.

In the beginning, the 9-Minute Perfect Mane routine will take you more than 9 minutes, and that is absolutely normal. With practice comes perfect, and your goal is to get better at grooming your curls in all of the 3 stages comprising your hair grooming routine. Give yourself plenty of time to get your hair grooming down to 9 minutes or less. Stay focused and aim to drop your hair grooming time slowly by following the 9-Minute Perfect Mane routine's template; eventually you will get to the 9-minute mark, all you need is some hands-on experience.

Most curly men complain about the time that it takes them to tame their waves, coils and kinks daily, yet the problem is not their curly hair, the problem is the way in which they approach their daily hair grooming. The way that I am showing you to approach your hair grooming is the tried and tested method to live in our modern day with a curly mane that is both aesthetic and convenient. We all want convenience without sacrificing cosmetic results, and, with the 9-Minute Perfect Mane routine, you will get the best of both worlds.

To illustrate how much you will benefit from this routine, I know ladies who spend 60 minutes on their hair before leaving the bathroom because the expert whom they read claims that doing so will give them superbly-defined fabulous curls. I also know plenty of curly men who just buzz their curls to a #1 every 2 weeks because they claim that it is impossible to manage their curly hair without spending a considerable amount of their morning working on their curls. Baloney, I say!

With the 9-Minute Perfect Mane routine and all the knowledge you have garnered so far, you will be able to get those curls looking the part while being able to devote all the time that you saved to either getting on time to work or doing manly stuff like hitting the gym hard and doing extracurricular bedroom activities. That's how I use my saved time, and that is how you should use it too!

Wrapping up your hair grooming routine

The 9-Minute Perfect Mane routine is a template that outlines the optimal order in which to base your cleaning, conditioning and styling stages. As laid out in the template, the 9-Minute Perfect Mane routine illustrates a typical shampooing day: you shampoo, then you condition, and then you move to styling your hair. Typically, your shampooing days will be longer than your non-shampooing days although the 9-Minute Perfect Mane routine is fully customisable according to your own needs and preferences.

Your hair grooming routine is always consistent in its sequence, goals, and emphasis on the 3 hair grooming main actions, but it will differ somewhat according to the day of the week as you remove or add secondary actions on each day; indeed, this adding and removing of secondary actions in your routine will depend, among other variables, on your shampooing frequency, conditioning frequency, a greater need for the Sebum Coating method or whether you want to style your hair or go solo (i.e. no hairstyling agent).

By now, you are ready to start creating your own hair grooming routine using the template for the 9-Minute Perfect Mane routine, adding or removing secondary actions on each day as you see fit, but, at all times, maintaining an emphasis on the main actions of cleaning, conditioning and styling.

For example, the Sebum Coating method has not been mentioned in the template for the 9-Minute Perfect Mane routine, but you know from reading this chapter that the Sebum Coating method is performed on your non-shampooing days, that the Sebum Coating method precedes the conditioning stage, that the Sebum Coating method has an inherent cleaning and conditioning action, and that the Sebum Coating method is the first secondary action that you implement on non-shampooing days. Furthermore, you can remove the conditioning stage on your non-shampooing days and be left with just the Sebum Coating method and the styling stage; you can even skip using any hairstyling agents for your mane and just do the Sebum Coating method, dry your curls and go hairstyle free on your non-shampooing days; it's that customisable!

I have attached in the Appendix (Appendix XXI) a table that illustrates what a hair grooming routine based on a 1 on/1 off shampooing frequency can look like when put into a week. It illustrates how each day has its own 9-Minute Perfect Mane routine albeit with variations in secondary actions while maintaining the focus on cleaning, conditioning and styling. The table also allows you to visualise the importance of having a hair grooming routine as you can see how each day of the week follows on to the next by taking into account what has been implemented the day before and what is to be implemented the day after.

The best way to create your hair grooming routine is to do so by building it around your shampooing frequency and using the template of the 9-Minute Perfect Mane routine on your shampooing days. Leave the conditioning frequency without experimenting until you find out your optimal shampooing frequency, and follow the initial guideline of only using a normal conditioner after the rinsing of the shampoo (i.e. on your shampooing days), then proceeding with the styling stage. Once you have sorted out your shampooing frequency, then you can start introducing the normal conditioner on your non-shampooing days as you desire.

On your non-shampooing days, start by using the Sebum Coating method, which does the cleaning and conditioning actions, then moving to the styling stage to be implemented with a leave-in conditioner and your chosen hairstyling agent. As it goes, the conditioning action on your non-shampooing days is provided by both the Sebum Coating method and the leave-in conditioner; the 3 stages and their main actions are satisfied because the Sebum Coating does the cleaning and conditioning while the leave-in also does the conditioning and provides the styling. What counts is that the sequence of the 3 main actions is respected so as to have an optimal hair grooming routine, whether it is a shampooing or non-shampooing day.

Going by the above, you can now see the importance of striving to find out your optimal shampooing frequency as your hair grooming routine is based around this hair-cleaning element. As you take the time to find out your optimal shampooing frequency, use the sequences of secondary actions for your shampooing and non-shampooing days that are illustrated below in Figure 21, and, once you have found out your optimal shampooing frequency, it is then that you can start customising the secondary actions to your desire such as increasing the frequency of use of normal and leave-in conditioners, using more hairstyling agents or inserting the Sebum Coating method on more days.

Figure 21 – Generic guidelines to start your hair grooming routine

STAGES	SHAMPOOING DAY	NON-SHAMPOOING DAY
Cleaning	Shampoo	Sebum Coating method
Conditioning	Normal conditioner	(dual action)
Styling	Yes	Yes
Leave-in conditioner?	No (style with other hairstyling agent)	Yes (style with leave-in + other hairstyling agent)

Overall, when you begin your awesome mane journey, stick to the initial guidelines of Figure 21 above for your shampooing and non-shampooing days and don't do any experiments with your secondary actions until you have secured your optimal shampooing frequency. Once secured, you can modify your routine but always abiding by the sequence of the hair grooming process and using a "trial and error" mindset in that if you experience regression of results, you must react promptly and undo any changes that have caused the regression.

Lastly, the same 3 tables in the Appendix (Appendix XXIII, Appendix XXIV and Appendix XXV) that I referenced at the beginning of this section have all the key elements of your hair grooming routine so that you can use a visual reference as you learn and apply all the content in this chapter. The tables are specific to the hair length categories and provide guidelines for everything concerning your hair grooming routine. It is now that you have finished this chapter that you can study these tables and understand them; thus, these tables are of special relevance when first setting up your hair grooming routine although any time that you modify your routine and find yourself having doubts, you can go back to the hair grooming guidelines in the tables as a new starting point.

My personal experience

It wasn't until I saw my hair grooming as a daily process consisting of 3 main actions and stages (cleaning, conditioning and styling) that I started making any real progress in my awesome mane journey. Once it was clear in my mind what the hair grooming process entailed, I was able to dig into and perfect each stage fully as I experimented with the secondary actions, finally achieving the necessary knowledge to create a successful and convenient hair grooming routine as the 9-Minute Perfect Mane routine is.

If you already know me from my site, you will be aware of how experimental I am. I have, for example, gone 30 days without using any products whatsoever (including no shampoo) on my long-length hair. I documented the experiment on my site, posting frequent updates, and the final cosmetic results were fantastic, considering that all I did was the Sebum Coating method for those 30 days. People from all over the world were coming to my site every day to see the updates and how I was progressing, and the consensus was that, indeed, my product-free hair experiment was successful.

While the above experiment was a bit extreme and risky as I only used water and the Sebum Coating method to groom my mane daily, I was able to prove that using shampoo daily is certainly not necessary for us curly men and that, if one knows his hair and uses the Sebum Coating method, one can go for lengthy periods of time without using shampoo or any other hair products (mind you, in an uber-minimalist manner, that is). Under usual and normal circumstances (i.e. no hair experiments!), however, my shampooing frequency is 1 on/6 off, and I have also used higher and lower shampooing frequencies for long periods of time as I adapted my frequency to my given life situation.

In terms of hair conditioners, I like to make my own kitchen-sink conditioners although I will also buy them online or off the supermarket shelf. I am a big believer in the frequent use of both normal and leave-in conditioners, and I like to use them concomitantly within the same hair grooming occasion: I will use the normal conditioner following the shampoo, and then I will use the leave-in as a hairstyling agent. Works like a charm and keeps my mane moisturised and tangle free.

On the other hand, I will sometimes rely on the Sebum Coating method as my only source of conditioner, only using a normal conditioner on the days that I shampoo. It really depends on how much time I have in the morning as the 9-Minute Perfect Mane routine is very time efficient and convenient on those days that I solely use the Sebum Coating method and go hairstyle free, and this natural cleaning and conditioning method still keeps my mane looking awesome without the need for artificial conditioners.

When it comes to styling curly hair, my eureka moment came when I decided to dump the hair brush that I was using. I kept wondering why my short curls looked like a ball of frizz despite I was brushing them like all those straight haired experts advised. Since I had nothing to lose and because I could always hit the barber and shave my curls if all failed, I decided to see what would happen if I dropped the hair brush for a few weeks and just styled my mane with my fingers. It turned out that dropping the hair brush was one of the best hair decisions that I have ever made, and, since then, I have not used a hair brush and instead use either my fingers or a wide-tooth comb for styling my hair. That was back in 2001, when the internet was still in an embryonic state for all male hair grooming matters.

With hairstyling agents, I switch them around as I deem appropriate, although I gravitate towards the natural styling approach of using blends of oils and even going solo without using hairstyling agents. I also like to use a leave-in conditioner as a hairstyling agent for that extra moisturising kick, and I especially use leave-ins as the foundation to other hairstyling agents that I may decide to use simultaneously (I'm a fan of styling creams and pomades). To dry my awesome mane, I do the Finger Shakeout when my curls are short, the conventional Shakeout when my curls are at medium length, and I use a cotton T-shirt and the conventional Shakeout when my curls are long.

As a whole, my hair grooming consists of the 9-Minute Perfect Mane routine with the secondary actions modified depending on my schedule and my current shampooing frequency. I use the same holistic hair grooming approach, routine and methods that I have given you in this chapter: I start with cleaning, follow with conditioning and finish with styling, adapting the secondary actions of each of the stages as the established schedule calls for, but always striving to clean, condition and style the hair daily. Throughout the years, I have found my hair grooming methodology, compiled into the 9-Minute Perfect Mane routine, to be the best for us curly men as it blends in convenience and flexibility with results, which is exactly what we, dudes with waves, coils and kinks, need to turn our curls into awesome manes!

4) Hair Care: Looking After Your Healthy Awesome Mane

"Learn to look after yourself"

A wise old man

In this chapter, I will cover how to keep your curly hair looking healthy and in optimal condition over the long term. While knowing your hair grooming and having a hair grooming routine is a must to get those curls looking awesome, you also need to address the optimal hair care of your mane in the long run, meaning that you must know the ins and outs of dealing with an awesome mane 24/7. Essentially, hair grooming yields instant cosmetic results while hair care yields cumulative cosmetic benefits and optimises the health aspect of your mane. Hair grooming and hair care go together in achieving an awesome mane, but it is important to have them separated and have a chapter dedicated to each so that you can see them as different key aspects of your awesome mane.

Having said all of the above, the use of the word "health" in this chapter is not literal. By "hair health", I will be referring to how your hair keeps its good looks in the long run, and the healthy and vigorous impression that it will exude. Have you ever taken a look at whatever cover dude is on the latest men's magazine and thought how his hair looked uber healthy? Apart from all the Photoshop retouching, it is not that his hair strands breathe in glorious amounts of oxygen or that his hair shafts are coated in nutritional blends engineered in some obscure laboratory. Nope, not even close; the dude just happens to know how to take care of his hair (that, or his image and PR teams know how to take care of his hair), thus his mane gets to look healthy.

Your hair can be made to look better, smoother and glossier (and thus, look "healthy") by not only grooming it properly but also by taking care of it when you go about your day-to-day business. Moreover, since hair doesn't have an ability to repair itself (as opposed to how skin does), the trick is to avoid damaging the hair in the first place, thus your hair care must have an special emphasis on preventing rather than fixing and should be seen as a strategy, for it will include a set of measures to be implemented long term.

With hair care, there is also a nutritional component that is of the utmost relevance and that is most commonly left out when men think of ways to look after their hair. Since the real living part of your hair is the follicle, the best hair care tactic to use so as to grow stronger and healthier-looking hair strands is to feed the follicle optimally; this is done via your nutritional approach: the sum of the foods you eat plus the nutritional supplements you may take. Altogether, the nutrients that you provide your body with via your nutritional approach nourish the tiny hair-producing factories that each hair follicle is. Considering that there are more than 100,000 follicles in the average male head, you've got some awesome nourishing to do!

Just like with hair grooming (and the rest of this book), I will too approach and show you all about the hair care and health of your awesome mane from the modern male perspective; convenience and long-term cosmetic results are the name of the game here.

The Big 3 awesome mane issues

As part of sporting an awesome mane, your daily hair care will be centred around preventing and addressing the following 3 issues:

1) Dry hair.

2) Tangled hair.

3) Hair loss (specifically, male pattern baldness).

You will encounter the first 2 on a daily basis, and the third one is included because hair loss is a serious issue that most men will experience sooner or later and that can be managed from the first day, even if you are not currently suffering from it.

Alone or in combination, these 3 issues have the potential to ruin the most optimally-groomed of all awesome manes, yet you must not be put off by these bad boys as they are issues that all males will experience, whether they have an awesome mane, a dead rat or simply want to tame the beast with a buzz cut. The good news is that a good hair care strategy will battle and minimise these issues while helping immensely in taking your curls to the next (awesome) level.

To fight these 3 issues on a daily basis, you have to think of hair care measures, and I have put these measures into 2 categories: proactive and reactive. Proactive measures imply actions that are taken to avoid issues happening in the first place while reactive measures imply actions that are taken to directly address the issue when it has happened. Proactive measures tend to be associated with the hair grooming process whereas reactive measures are part of a more ad hoc approach, for you will be performing your reactive measures to fix a problem instead of purposely preventing it as with proactive measures.

The emphasis placed on these proactive and reactive measures will become more important as you grow your mane into the medium and long lengths. Near-shaved and short curly hair can get away with skipping some of the hair care measures or not being as careful, but I highly recommend you to follow all described measures regardless of your hair length if you want to ensure the never-ending optimal health of your awesome mane.

As men with curly hair, it isn't just what we do in the bathroom that matters. Once we step outside, we must also keep an eye on our manes because our curly hair is curly the 24 hours of the day, hence you must think like a curly man 24/7. Through my years of experimenting, banging my head against the wall and shaving my head only to grow my curls again, I have been able to come up with these proactive and reactive hair care measures specific to each of our awesome mane issues.

Dry hair

Battling this bad boy is your main goal when it comes to hair care. Dry hair is easy to identify as it feels like hay, is frizzy and brittle, and the curls are not defined. The opposite of dry hair is moisturised hair: curls feel light and smooth, look more defined and are much easier to manage. Do not confuse, however, dry hair with drying your hair: the latter is part of your hair grooming routine and aims to remove excess water from the hair so as to leave it damp (thus, with moisturise), whereas the former (dry hair) is hair that has been stripped of moisture and is the result of improper hair care and a subpar hair grooming routine.

I always say this, if you can keep your hair from losing its moisture and becoming dry in the first place, you will have solved 99% of your awesome mane worries. Curly hair, as we already know, is naturally predisposed to being dry due to its curving nature, and this predisposition increases the higher up we go in the curl type range. This is just how it is, and it is part of the territory of having curly hair. Dry hair is brittle and frizzy, and the locks will interlock (i.e. tangle) easily, which is exactly the opposite of what makes an awesome mane.

Luckily for us, there are hair care measures, both proactive and reactive, that will put an end to dry hair. Dry hair takes days to manifest if it is occurring from an awesome mane (i.e. moisturised curls), so you will be able to notice daily in the mirror how your hair slowly becomes dry, thus allowing you to tackle this issue before it gets really bad.

Proactive:

- Go easy on very hot environments. This means saunas, very hot showers or extreme temperatures (think desert type). As a modern male, it is impossible to avoid these environments unless you want to live a life of boredom so just don't go crazy on them, especially saunas (e.g. don't hit the sauna for extended periods of time on a daily basis).

- Stop shampooing every day. Drop your shampooing frequency; really aim to find your optimal frequency as described in the previous hair grooming chapter. This measure works rapidly and extremely well to prevent the risk of your hair becoming dry.

- Use a leave-in conditioner for much of your hair grooming efforts. Try to change your hairstyles to those that are optimally styled with a leave-in alone or in conjunction with other hairstyling agents (apply the leave-in conditioner first). Hairstyles that are favoured by leave-in conditioners are those where the hair doesn't have to be held in a gravity-defying position.

- Do not blow-dry your hair on a daily basis. If you want to use a hair dryer (i.e. blow-dry your hair), clip a diffuser to it, coat your hair priorly with a heat-protecting hair product and use the coldest temperature available in the settings. Furthermore, never blow-dry wet or soaked hair, only blow-dry your hair when it is damp.

- Use a normal conditioner after shampooing, and, once you have your optimal shampooing frequency worked out, play with increasing your conditioning frequency. Normal conditioners only take 2 minutes to be left on as you continue to shower, and, if you master the 9-Minute Perfect mane routine, your busiest hair grooming day will take less than 9 minutes.

- Aim to wet your hair every day, regardless of whether it is a shampooing or non-shampooing day. Water plus your sebum and/or an artificial conditioner equates moisturised hair strands.

- Do not alter your curls: don't straighten them, bleach them or do anything to permanently alter their texture or structure. Altering your hair will damage it, weaken it and make it more prone to dryness. It will also destroy your natural curl pattern, making it harder to have defined curls.

Reactive:

- If you currently have hair that has been straightened permanently, or if you have been using hair-straightening gadgets (e.g. flat irons), it is a good idea to start from a fresh batch of hair. Cut your hair and start growing new hair that will now be managed as an awesome mane.

- When you find your hair starting to look dry, schedule a normal conditioner session (i.e. the secondary action of using a normal conditioner) as soon as possible. It can be on the same day or a few days later, just don't delay it for more than 3 days.

- Shampoo before the scheduled conditioner session, then don't shampoo again for the next 7 days. After the stipulated 7-day period of no shampooing, go back to your usual shampooing frequency.

- For the next 7 days after you initially address your dry hair, use a normal conditioner on every day and hit the leave-in conditioner extra hard on all 7 days (i.e. use it every day and in copious amounts).

- Make sure to also do the Sebum Coating method every day for these 7 days (remember, the Sebum Coating method is always the first secondary action).

- If you are starting your awesome mane journey with very dry hair, I advise you to use a deep conditioner every 2 weeks for the next 8 weeks. Deep conditioners are stronger forms of normal conditioners, and you will find them next to normal conditioners in wherever it is that you buy your hair products from. You can also use a hair mask instead of a deep conditioner if you so prefer.

Tangled hair

Your hair will tangle and form knots, that's a reality. Together with dry hair, the sooner you accept and face this fact, the sooner you will get your awesome mane of curls. Just like with dry hair, tangled hair is best managed with proactive measures because curls can tangle very bad, to the point that the tangled mess has to be chopped. Tangled hair can actually form hair knots that are, to put it bluntly, evil. I have experienced some cunningly formed knots over the years that I had to ultimately chop as I perfected my proactive measures although nowadays I got so good at it that I seldom get an evil tangled lock (I normally get them when I do experiments). For the record, chopping a tangle or hair knot should always be the last resort, always!

Generally, the higher-end your curl type is, the more its propensity to tangle will be and having dry hair will further magnify your risk of tangling. Thus, keeping your mane moisturised and dry free is in itself a great proactive measure, but it will not totally protect you from developing some nasty tangles, hence you need to emphasise your tangled-hair proactive measures at all costs. Moreover, an excess build up of sebum or hairstyling agents can cause your curls to tangle too, thus the importance of finding out and having an optimal shampooing frequency.

Curly hair will also tend to tangle more the longer it is. Expect to have to put yourself to use with this "tangling" matter on a frequent basis once your curls hit a long length. If you want to grow your awesome mane to a long length and beyond, be prepared to find a few tangles every day despite your proactive efforts. That's the nature of the beast!

Once you find a tangled lock of hair, you must approach the detangling task like a surgeon would approach an operation, which is why I truly want you to see cutting the tangled hair as a last measure: a good surgeon never gives up on his patient! Detangling is in itself an art, and the more you practise it, the better you will get at it, just like with hair grooming.

Detangling requires you to softly pull the length of the hair that precedes the tangle or knot and use a pulling motion that goes towards the direction of the scalp. You must use plenty of conditioner or natural oils to grease the tangle priorly, which means that detangling is just an awful and messy procedure altogether and is best avoided. Thus, fellow curly head, you must do all within reach to work your proactive measures hard. Be aware that some of the following measures are a bit annoying, and it is up to you whether you want to apply them or not; ultimately, the more you use them, the better your mane will look.

Proactive:

- Run your fingers through your hair strands every time that you use a normal conditioner. Apply the conditioner to your hair, and run your fingers or wide-tooth comb from the scalp down the tips. You can do this measure as you see fit, for you can do it during the 2 minutes that the normal conditioner has to be left on the hair (conditioning stage) and you can also do it when you are applying the leave-in conditioner (styling stage). Unlike in the Sebum Coating method where your fingers are placed in a pinching manner, you run your fingers through your curls to detangle with your fingers forming a rake, which essentially mimics a wide-tooth comb. Thus, either use your fingers or a wide-tooth comb for this proactive measure.

- Tie your curls when you go to bed. This is only applicable to those with medium or long-length curls. Secure your locks into a ponytail or, better yet, into a bun or braid. Use a hair band, do not use any rubber band you find around. If the length of your mane is not enough to tie all of the hair into one bun, then don't be afraid to tie your hair into 2, 3 or even 4 buns. Just warn anyone who may see you the next morning when you wake up (you can skip this measure for one-night stands!).

- If your hair is of a short length, then you can use a dorag or sleeping hair cap to secure your mane and avoid the hair being loose. While sleeping caps are traditionally associated with women and weird hair potions, sleeping caps are secretly used by quite a good portion of men who know of the sleeping cap's benefits in avoiding tangled hair. I have used them in the past though for the most part I prefer to go solo (i.e. no hair cap) if my hair is short.

- For bedtime, I also recommend you to sleep on pillow cases made of satin or silk. The former is not very expensive and will help prevent your mane from tangling at night. Silk is very comfortable and smooth to have your head resting on but is obviously the more expensive option. These 2 types of fabric reduce the friction on your hair from rubbing your head on the pillow as you sleep, which aids greatly in discouraging the tangling of your locks.

- Use a leave-in conditioner most of the time for your styling. Not only is this hairstyling agent great for adding extra conditioning to your locks but it is also great for adding extra slip to your curls and avoiding the risk of tangling. Apply the leave-in first and then apply your other chosen hairstyling agents.

- When drying your mane, avoid using a conventional towel. Use a 100% cotton T-shirt instead, and you can do like me and buy a few cheap ones, which you'll use solely for drying your hair. If you use a conventional towel, do as I recommend in the previous chapter and smoothly pass the towel over your curls as you squeeze them; never rub the towel vigorously against your hair as this is a sure way to get your hair frizzy and tangled in an instant! There are also some bath towels that don't have rough surfaces, and you can use this type of towels if you'd rather dry your hair with a towel than with a T-shirt.

- Tie your mane on windy days. If you cannot tie your curls, use plenty of leave-in conditioner before you leave the house. Same goes for driving a convertible car, tie your hair or use a leave-in conditioner. I still remember when I took a lady out in my convertible early into my awesome mane journey: I started the date with my mane looking great, and, by the end of the drive, I was sporting a full-on dead rat atop my head. Lesson learnt, tie your curls or use a leave-in conditioner if you are going to be in a windy environment.

- Avoid unnecessarily rubbing your head against surfaces such as head rests or couches. This one is a bit excessive, and, if you can't be bothered to use this measure, at least tie your hair if you have medium/long-length curls. For example, I would tie my medium-length curls every time that I would go for long car rides.

- Once your curls get to hang down, try to keep the hair tied for a good portion of your day. The more the hair is hanging down and dangling, the more the chances of tangling.

Reactive:

- Tackle a tangle/knot as soon as you spot it. The longer you wait, the worse it will get.

- Before detangling, use either a normal conditioner or a natural oil to coat the tangle and provide slip. Don't only coat the tangle, coat the whole lock of hair in which the tangle is found. Coconut oil and olive oil work great as natural oils to provide slip.

- When detangling, pull softly the tangled hair towards the scalp with one hand as you pinch the tangle/knot firmly with the other hand. It is preferable that you use your fingers for this measure instead of a wide-tooth comb; the wide-tooth comb is best used as a rake for your proactive measures.

- If the tangle is big and you find it hard to detangle, pour apple cider vinegar on the tangle and leave the vinegar on the tangle without rinsing for 5 minutes. One of the reasons for tangles to form is due to an overaccumulation of sebum that has hardened; the apple cider vinegar works to soften the sebum, allowing for better detangling. After the stipulated 5 minutes, rinse the vinegar, and then coat the tangle with normal conditioner or oil to continue detangling.

- Chopping is the last option; even very bad tangles can be fixed with patience, and you can work them in separate sessions instead of in a single session. You may find at times, however, a tangle so viciously formed that you will just have to chop it off. Weigh the pros and cons of doing this and remember that the tangled hair will continue to tangle more and more if you don't do anything about it immediately. Sometimes, you will just have to give up on your follicular patient!

- Once you have detangled the lock, wet it and coat it with normal conditioner. If you had to work through several tangles in that session, soak all of your hair in water and apply normal conditioner to all of your mane. Rinse the conditioner as usual after 2 minutes, then apply a leave-in conditioner to the hair. Resume your hair grooming schedule the next day.

Hair loss

This one is a big issue for us men, and there are 2 main forms of hair loss that you will be facing with an awesome mane: shedding and balding.

Shedding is a natural scalp process in which a given hair strand detaches itself from the scalp while the rest of hair strands in the scalp continue to grow. Shedding is part of a healthy follicle's life cycle, and each hair strand in your scalp has an expiration date; at the end of the hair's life cycle, the hair strand simply detaches itself, making room in the follicle for a new hair strand to grow from scratch. On average, males shed approximately 100 hair strands per day, and you will notice a lot of shed hairs in the shower or everywhere in the house once you start taking good care of your hair.

When one doesn't groom his curls properly, one carries around plenty of shed hairs that are, in fact, trapped in the waves, coils or kinks of one's dead rat, meaning that those shed hairs haven't actually fallen off yet, despite being effectively detached from the hair follicles. It is once you start using conditioners and keeping your curls optimally coated with sebum that you will start seeing more hairs falling off than usual. Do not worry; this is completely normal as your moisturised curls will now have more slip and the shed hairs will be allowed to fall off instead of remaining trapped in your mane's curves. The visibility of your shed hairs will also be exacerbated if you grow your curls to a medium or long length (the longer your hair is, the more visible the shed hairs will be).

The other relevant form of hair loss is balding: a hair loss process that is not part of the healthy life cycle of a hair strand (as opposed to hair shedding) and that can be caused by several factors including one's genes, certain medications, stress, disease or hormones. To us men, the most important form of balding is male pattern baldness (MPB); the form of permanent balding that men experience due to being, well, men!

Your body as a male produces several sex hormones, and one of them, dihydrotestosterone (DHT), is one of the culprits behind MPB. Dihydrotestosterone is responsible for giving you your masculine attributes (e.g. a deep voice or thick hair covering your body), but it also has the negative effect of slowly killing away your hair follicles if you are predisposed to MPB. The MPB process is not fully understood, but research points to DHT and inherited genes being two of the key pieces in the MPB puzzle. For what is worth, your own unique genetic response to DHT is what will ultimately predispose you to MPB; just because you have high levels of DHT, it doesn't mean that you will go bald.

Male pattern baldness is a slow process that is actually classified in stages so as to gauge its evolution. The most common scale used is the Hamilton-Norwood scale pioneered by Dr. James Hamilton in the '50s, and later revised by Dr. O'Tar Norwood in the '70s. Also simplified and known as the Norwood scale, this staging method classifies MPB in 7 progressive stages starting with recession of the forehead's hairline towards the vertex and increased frontal hair thinning (Stage I to II), and finishing with no hair at all on the top and back of the head (Stage VII). Since MPB will commonly begin at both sides of the forehead's hairline (i.e. the temples), it is easy for MPB to go unnoticed in its initial stages; this being the reason behind my emphasis on keeping a close eye on one's hairline if MPB runs in the family. I recommend you to fully research the topic of male pattern baldness as there are some good online and offline resources to learn from, and it is imperative for you to see a good dermatologist or medical specialist if you suspect MPB.

For our third issue of hair loss, I will give you the proactive and reactive measures to primarily guard yourself against MPB although you will also find some lifestyle choices that will help towards preventing not only MPB but also hair loss attributed to stress and other external factors. With regards to hair shedding, you have nothing to worry about as, again, it is a completely natural process.

Proactive:

- If MPB runs in your family and you are over the age of 18, start taking photos of your hairline. Take pictures every 3 months of the front, top, side and back of your head. If MPB doesn't run in your family, yet you are concerned about losing your hair, take pictures every 6 months instead. Compare the pictures that you have taken over time: any receding at the temples and lowered hair density that is noticed is a sign of MPB.

- Since MPB has a strong inherited component, do some family investigation and try to speak to family members to know which males in the family line have gone bald and at what age (go back a few generations). Contrary to popular belief, MPB can be passed from both the maternal and the paternal lineage, not just the mother's side as the myth goes. Also, if any males in the last 2 generations of your family tree have gone bald before the age of 35, it will mean that there is a strong MPB predisposition in the family so keep a close eye on your hair as advised in the previous point.

- Read as much as you can on MPB. Be aware, however, that the hair loss industry is full of scammers and snake oil products. Keep an eye on my site among other sources for trusted content on MPB.

- If you tie your hair, make sure to not tie it tight. When you tie your hair, release tension from the follicles by slightly and smoothly pulling the tied hair against the

(follows from previous page)

direction of the ponytail/bun/braid. You can actually lose hair from leaving your hair tied too tight, with this form of hair loss being known as "traction alopecia".

- Totally avoid hair brushes and conventional/pocket combs. As I have emphasised in the styling section of the previous chapter "Hair Grooming: Get Those Curls Looking Great", only use your fingers or a wide-tooth comb to style your curls. Hair brushes and combs will have you pulling your curls excessively, which will damage the hair strands and follicles.

- If your hair shedding is getting out of hand, start keeping a close eye on your hairline as well as on the hair density on top of your head. Intense emotional stress or distraught can bring about a temporary increase in hair shedding, and the hair loss will not follow the predictable temple recession of MPB. In any case, monitor your hairline and hair density as MPB is the form of hair loss that is most relevant to you, for it is irreversible.

- Avoid hairstyles that have you pulling your hair too hard, such as excessively side parting your curls so that your hair looks straightened. Again, avoid any excessive pulling of your hair and choose hairstyles that do not require you to manipulate your curls too much especially if you already suffer from MPB.

- Make sure that your diet is spot on. This means eating a healthy diet emphasising a good amount of protein and fish oils as well as an optimal intake of micronutrients (i.e. minerals and vitamins). This chapter contains a section on what to look for in order to build an awesome-mane-friendly diet.

- Exercise improves blood circulation, and one of the theories explaining MPB goes that this form of hair loss is partially caused by an inadequate supply of blood flow to the hair follicles. While it would be a wild exaggeration to directly link exercising with the curing of MPB, it will not do you any damage to exercise frequently so that you pair an awesome mane with an awesome and healthy body. If exercising does provide a benefit to male pattern baldness (however small the benefit may be), then you'll at least have killed 2 birds with 1 stone!

- I know it sounds easier said than done but try to minimise high levels of chronic stress. Chronic stress not only exacerbates hair loss but it also makes you age faster and decreases your quality of life. Ask yourself, does this added stress bring a benefit to any area of my life? Life is about balance, harmony and taking actions, so carefully analyse and evaluate the pros and cons of living your life with high levels of stress.

- Research your medications. There are many medications that list hair loss as a side effect and concomitant use of medications that can cause hair loss complicates matters even more. Always read the medication's warnings, and it is in your interest to always check with your doctor the potential side effects of any new medication that you are put on. Likewise, if you are having to take a medication for the long term and are experiencing hair loss, talk to your doctor so as to be able to know whether the hair loss is being induced by the medication or if you are suffering from MPB.

- Have blood panels performed once a year. I do this myself for optimal health, and it will allow you to build up a log of how your body is performing throughout a given time period of your life. It will also help you to potentially identify anything that is going wrong. Test your thyroid, sex hormones, glucose levels and stress hormones for a direct link to hair loss if any of these are subpar. Speak to your doctor for the best approach to perform blood tests on a yearly basis. Be aware though, it can get expensive.

Reactive:

- If you have noticed your hairline receding, see a dermatologist as soon as possible. If he/she confirms MPB and you want to slow down the hair loss progression, then go on minoxidil, a drug that is almost free of side effects and that works best in the earlier stages of MPB. I must tell you, however, that there is no cure for male pattern baldness as of 2013.

- Finasteride is another proven-to-work medication, but it can have some heavy side effects in some users. I recommend you to not only see a dermatologist but also an endocrinologist if you decide to take finasteride. Get an initial blood panel measuring your hormone levels (especially levels of sex hormones), and re-test on a frequent basis as recommended by your doctor. Finasteride works by inhibiting an enzyme that converts testosterone into DHT, hence the use of finasteride should be monitored for optimal male health.

- There are other substances that may work to treat male pattern baldness, but you are best seeking the advice of a dermatologist with regards to these experimental substances. Unfortunately, many of these substances are being pushed by scammers, giving a bad image to potential substances that could work to treat MPB. Among these potentially-helpful substances are ketoconazole, saw palmetto, topical caffeine, tea tree oil, several vitamins and mineral and other natural alternatives. Do always remain skeptic of anything making wild claims; the only medications clinically-approved to treat MPB as of 2013 are minoxidil and finasteride (though dutasteride has shown great promise and may be approved at some stage).

- A hair transplant is a feasible option for those males who want to get their hair back. However, it is imperative that you research this option thoroughly because transplanting hair is a very skilled process. Furthermore, a hair transplant doesn't guarantee 100% that the transplanted hair will be MPB free, and a good hair transplant will cost thousands of dollars and will typically require more than one session.

- If you have just pulled out a chunk of hair accidentally (it will happen eventually if you grow your mane to a long length), massage the area immediately for 30 seconds, ingest 100 milligrams of vitamin C and move on. Hair that is pulled out of its follicle socket will grow back eventually, but don't make pulling out your hair a habit because repeatedly plucking your hair will damage the follicle and irreversibly halt its production of hair material (i.e. no more growth of hair strands).

- If you find yourself experiencing hair loss because you keep pulling out your hair, see a doctor. This hair-pulling habit is known as trichotillomania in the medical field and is associated with chronically-high levels of stress, anxiety and even some mental disorders. Tackling the root of the problem (no pun intended) will fix this cause of hair loss. Be aware that trichotillomania is not only limited to scalp hair, it can be manifested on other areas of the body (the eyebrow is a common area). In its most extreme form, trichotillomania will lead to bald patches in the scalp.

A note on how overall health reflects on hair health

I have decided to include this section in this hair-health-oriented chapter because, as modern males, we should care for our overall health too.

Listen; men live about 5 years less than women, and we go about our lives with a lot of unneeded stress and drama. Ultimately, our overall health will reflect on our hair health just as it will reflect on our sexual health or mental health.

As you have read in the previous section with regards to hair loss, this third awesome mane issue is a serious condition linked with stress and hormones. A stressed body produces more cortisol, distorts its release of growth hormone and insulin, and decreases its levels of sex hormones, with all of this in unison enhancing and magnifying any hair loss taking place.

Biologically, when the body is under extreme physical or mental demands for long periods (i.e. chronic stress), it will shut down several unnecessary-to-life processes so as to remain efficient and ensure survival. Your body will prioritise your brain before your hair follicles when it is in survival mode, which is why people who are overstressed or malnourished experience dramatic hair loss and don't look good physically. On top of that, stressed people tend to be depressed, and depression is a serious health condition that will negatively impact your desire to look good including the grooming and looking after of your hair.

Let's be real, though. Avoiding all sources of stress is not possible, and, in fact, some additional stress can be good for you as it makes you have to think more as well as learn and adapt to dynamic environments. As a modern-day male, you will go through bouts of high stress during your life; it just isn't feasible to live a stress-free life unless you consider moving to some Tibetan monastery so as to spend your remaining days as a monk (and I still have my doubts of that working 100%!).

If you find yourself constantly going through periods of high stress and can't see the light, stop. Stop right now. Take a big breath and sit back. Think.

Many times, we men just get carried away with the monotony of life, conforming to whatever we are spoon-fed and avoiding thinking outside the box. We sacrifice long-term happiness for short-term rewards and, in the process, throw our lives out of balance. I know that having $10,000 flowing into your bank account every last day of the month may be awesome, but how are you going to spend it if you don't have the time to even meet the right partner or make true friends instead of social acquaintances? Or how about busting your derriere at work so as to be able to send your kids to the best schools, yet only getting to see them in their sleep as you come home from work at 11 every single night?

I am no one to tell you what you should do and what you should not do with your life. In fact, this book is about opening your eyes so that you get to view your curly hair as another integral element of your life and finally embrace something that is inherent to you. I can only go so far in this book to give you the best advice that I can with regards to your hair; at the end of the day, it is you who makes his decisions and takes actions based on acquired knowledge and proper evaluation. Just like with your hair, I would like for you to be the best you can, hence the reason for my emphasis on weighting the pros and cons of any added stress to your life because going through life in a miserable manner is a great way to waste one's life. Stop, think, process, evaluate and be proud of the actions that you decide to take and implement.

If you are one of those men experiencing too much stress in his life or who cannot handle his current piling of life stresses, look for help. There is nothing emasculating or girly about seeking out help. Real men think positive and take assertive actions so as to find the best ways to benefit themselves and their loved ones. Someone who is overstressed and cannot enjoy life will not only drag himself down but also those who surround him. You've already paved the way by deciding to acquire your awesome mane, all you need now is to milk the momentum, and I trust that, were you to currently find yourself in a dark period of your life, you will break through and continue to walk a life full of successes with your awesome mane, my friend.

Optimising nutrition for an awesome mane

You may have heard before the saying "you are what you eat". While I don't wholeheartedly agree with this cliché, I have seen on myself and on others what optimal nutrition can do to one's hair and even life. From better curls to a better body to an overall better life, your nutrition should be optimised to cater to your lifestyle as a 21st century male.

"Organic", "fat-free", "Atkins diet", "free of preservatives", "no-carb pizza" or "aspartame" are just some of the fancy words that we get bombarded with every day. For the most part, we don't know what they are or what they really mean, and unfortunately we have to live with the fact that many companies and people out there take advantage of semantic boundaries and wrongful associations. Organic food is twice as expensive as non-organic food, yet being organic doesn't guarantee it to be healthier or diet friendly as many people wrongfully think of organic foods. Likewise, low-fat products are not necessarily healthier than their regular counterparts, and, many times, the fat content of the former is substituted by adding lots of sugar and other just as unhealthy ingredients (e.g. high-fructose corn syrup) to mask the food's otherwise bland taste. In fact, next time that you are in the supermarket, go to the dairy section and read the ingredients of the flashiest and most-colourful low-fat yoghurt that you can find on display, and see this nutritional dichotomy for yourself.

Over the years, I have found that whatever diet I chose that improved my health also had the side effect of improving my hair. The body is a perfect machine relying on homeostasis and biological harmony, hence a change in one bodily process will have a knock-on effect on other bodily processes, and thus the need to see one's diet as a way to improve one's health and body as a whole and, by default, one's hair. What's more is that an optimal diet and nutritional approach will not only improve the looks of your awesome mane but also ensure that your hair remains atop your head for a long time.

Your hair follicles are alive, and, for them to produce hair, they need optimal nutrition as well as blood flow to deliver the right nutrients. Your hair follicles are dug in your skin, the latter (skin) being the largest organ in the body, so a lot of internal processes are going on to allow the hair follicles to continue to produce hair material (i.e. hair strands) non-stop. Thus, while throwing exotic ingredients on your hair strands in the hopes that your hair can breathe more oxygen or can live happily is an exercise in futility, there is certainly quite a merit and good sense in trying to get optimal nutrients delivered to your hair follicles endogenously (i.e. via your diet and nutritional approach).

There is no one-and-only nutritional approach to making your hair look its best. In my case, the nutritional approach that I have used successfully, and which I will share with you, is one that I have found to allow for optimal sebum secretion, a healthy scalp, stronger and thicker hair strands, and is one that has also helped me to avoid excessive hair shedding or being hit by male pattern baldness. The aforementioned benefits brought by my optimal nutritional approach have greatly promoted the good looks and optimal health of my mane, and, so far, it has allowed me to secure my awesome mane for the long term as I have paired my nutritional approach with a solid set of proactive and reactive hair care measures (i.e. my tailored hair care strategy).

There are a lot of diets out there and plenty of nutritional approaches that one can follow. Through my experience, I have found a positive correlation between my overall health and the health of my hair: whenever my health was at its peak via my nutritional approach, so was my hair's health. Thus, the nutritional approach that I follow is my 1 stone to kill 2 juicy birds: optimal overall health and optimal hair health.

What is a nutritional approach? That which comprises everything you ingest, from the foods you eat (i.e. diet) to the nutritional supplements you may so take, altogether providing you with macronutrients (protein, carbohydrates and fats) and micronutrients (vitamins, minerals and other essential nutrients) that are used by the body to support its functioning and to maintain your health and well-being. In the context of this book, your nutritional approach is made up of your diet and your nutritional supplementation (the latter being optional).

When it comes to your diet, you should not be seeing it as a short-term change in your nutritional habits in order to lose weight or look better. Instead, your diet should be integrated into a nutritional approach seeking optimal health above all as, in turn, such a diet will enhance your hair and image. This has been exactly my case, which is why I want to include and share in this chapter my nutritional approach for an awesome mane so that you can learn about an indispensable element to having great hair that is overlooked by the majority of men desiring better hair.

The diet that I follow is high in protein intake, low in carbohydrate intake and moderate in fat intake. After years of experimenting with different ratios of these 3 macronutrients (protein:carbohydrates:fats), I have found such "high protein:low carbohydrate:moderate fat" diet to be the best for me and for my hair. I also try to eat as close to natural as possible, so I always choose the least-processed and man-modified food items, which automatically ensures that I get the most amount of nutrients from the foods I eat. An example of this would be orange juice: instead of buying a pack of processed orange juice from the supermarket shelf, I will instead buy oranges in their natural state and then make the orange juice myself. I apply this very principle to my diet and when I buy food; that way I am guaranteed to maximise the food that I eat from both a nutritional and economical perspective.

I have not only seen this on myself but on others too: a diet composed of a high protein, low carbohydrate and moderate fat intake, together with a natural and unprocessed food emphasis is the best dietary option to safeguard one's awesome mane over the long term. My hair has looked its best with a diet like this one, and I have been able to notice the changes in the health and looks of my hair when I have gone back to using such a diet at different points in my lifetime. If we consider this diet's documented health benefits and the huge anecdotal evidence that can be found online vouching for a natural and unprocessed diet, it then leaves no doubt that a diet similar to mine is a great addition for the health-conscious modern male who wants to achieve and maintain his awesome mane.

It is thus that I would like to give you the insight to my diet and nutritional approach so that you can learn from what has worked for me and then be able to apply some of my nutritional principles and tactics to your awesome mane journey. As a cautionary note, I must warn you that you should at all times consult a doctor before embarking on a diet regimen (including mine) or doing anything that may affect your health in one way or another. Your health should always come first no matter what, so first consult with your doctor if you decide to change your dietary habits or emulate my personal experience with my nutritional approach for optimal hair health.

My diet

I only eat once or twice a day on average. I prefer to avoid spiking my insulin levels frequently because I don't like the consequent fluctuations in blood sugar levels. I feel that my optimal energy levels are best achieved with fasting for the most part of my day, and I prefer to enjoy 1 or 2 big meals instead of snacking throughout the day.

I also stick to certain food groups that I have found to be the essentials for overall health and hair health. I reward myself with eating whatever I want once every 1 or 2 weeks (i.e. a cheat day); I'll do this typically on a Friday or Saturday as this is when it is most convenient for a social life. I prefer not to obsess about breaking my diet, and I will break my diet if the occasion calls for it, then making up for it by either exercising more or delaying the next cheat day. Regardless, 90% of my time is spent either fasted or eating from the food groups below:

- Meat: lean cuts and from the butcher. I avoid processed meat for the most part. Steak and chicken breast make a big chunk of my meat intake, and I love eating them. I also gulp down whole chickens often, there is just something primitive and manly about devouring 2 whole chickens with your hands in one sitting. I throw in some vegetables with the 2 chickens for an added healthy touch (cavemen also ate their veggies). High-quality protein is of the utmost value to grow strong hair strands, and meat (be it red or white) provides high quantities of high-quality protein as well as hair-friendly micronutrients such as zinc and several B vitamins.

- Oily fish: I eat salmon or sardines at least once a week. Canned sardines are my favourite and despite their light processing to fit inside the can, they still remain very nutritious and are very tasty in extra-virgin olive oil. With salmon, I prefer to oven cook it or fry it lightly with slow heat. The precious nutrients that I seek in oily fish are omega-3 fatty acids, which are essential fats needed for optimal sebum production. Most oily fishes also contain vitamin A, which is an excellent skin moisturiser and sustains optimal skin cell production (i.e. optimises the health of your hair follicles).

- Dairy: I love cheese, and I eat cheese regularly. I prefer the unpasteurised type because it is made with raw milk (less processing): good Manchego (Spanish),

(follows from previous page)

Parmesan (Italian) and Emmental (Swiss) cheeses are made with unpasteurised milk and taste great. I also eat a good amount of cottage cheese and yoghurt; I don't drink much milk because I find that it gives me too much stomach discomfort if I drink more than 2 pints. Dairy is another excellent source of high-quality protein and also provides many hair-friendly vitamins including vitamin A and the many Bs.

- Eggs: I call eggs "nature's multivitamin". They are a staple in my diet, and I strive to eat 2 to 6 whole eggs per day. After experimenting with different quantities, I have found a relatively-high daily consumption of eggs to have absolutely no negative effect on my cholesterol levels. Eggs have so many nutrients that are essential to male health (including hair health) that leaving them out of one's diet should be regarded as nutritional suicide. They are also cheap and multifunctional, and I eat them mostly boiled or scrambled.

- Fruits: I base most of my fruit intake around berries and water-dense fruits such as pomegranates and kiwis. They are packed with a wide array of nutrients and antioxidants not found elsewhere in nature, so I consider these fruits essential to optimal health and hair.

- Vegetables: I go through pounds of leafy vegetables every week, and I eat most leafy veggies. I also eat tomatoes, cucumbers and onions every day, and I make salads with all of these plus the leafy vegetables. I do not eat starchy vegetables except for the occasional beetroot. Most vegetables contain ample amounts of hair-essential vitamin C and antioxidants.

- Water: I drink tap water except if I am living in a country with bad-quality tap water (e.g. Dubai). I drink about 3 litres of water per day and go through an extra 3 litres in each weightlifting session that I carry out. I find that most people, including myself, overeat when they are thirsty because the body activates the hunger cue so as to obtain water from food sources since it is not getting it from liquid sources. Sipping water throughout the day is a great way to kill any unneeded hunger pangs, and I have a big glass of water sitting next to me as I type these words. Adequate and daily internal hydration (i.e. drinking water) is indispensable to life, including skin health (and by default your hair follicles).

- Oils: I only use extra-virgin olive oil for cooking and dressing because not only is this oil resistant to heat but it is also packed with vitamin E and monounsaturated fat, so this particular oil doesn't alter my intake ratio of omega-3:omega-6 fatty acids (as opposed to how sunflower oil would do). Despite being the most expensive of oils, I always buy extra-virgin olive oil from Spain since southern Spain has the best region in the world to grow olives, and the olive oil from there is magnificent. Always go "extra-virgin" because it is the least refined (processed) of oils and contains the highest levels of vitamin E, a vitamin that behaves as an antioxidant in the body and that has a skin-enhancing effect.

- Nuts: at least once a week, I eat a blend of almonds, pecan nuts and walnuts. Just like with extra-virgin olive oil, nuts are a great source of vitamin E and are tasty. I like to use them in salads because they make salads taste great and you can get creative with them. Since vitamin E is a liposoluble vitamin (i.e. the body stores it), you don't need to eat nuts every day: once or twice a week is sufficient for a hair-friendly intake of vitamin E.

- Fats: I also use butter from milk as well as extra-virgin coconut butter. The butter I use is from cows that have grazed in grass since grass-fed cows produce higher-quality milk. I buy extra-virgin coconut butter because not only is it great for hair as a hairstyling agent but also because it is a great cooking butter if I decide to cook something exotic. Butter contains vitamin A, which is the big daddy of hair-friendly micronutrients.

- Iodised salt: I use iodised salt because most foods lack in iodine. Iodine is a nutrient that is of the utmost importance for the proper functioning of the thyroid gland. A low intake of iodine will manifest in the body as hair loss and brittle hair, apart from causing other hypothyroid-like symptoms. Iodised salt is an excellent way to fulfil one's daily intake of iodine.

All of the above foods are what I would eat on a weekly basis. I pick and rotate them daily so as to meet my macronutrient and micronutrient needs and have variety in my diet. My fridge is always full of these food items, and I try to avoid precooked food because I want to know what I am putting in my mouth.

My supplementation

While I don't always use nutritional supplements, I like to use them frequently so as to complement my diet and bulletproof my nutritional approach. On a daily basis, I typically add the following nutrients in the form of supplements to my diet:

- Calcium.

- Magnesium.

- Zinc.

- Copper.

- Vitamin B complex.

- Multivitamin with 100% of the Reference Daily Intake (RDI).

- Vitamin C with rose hips.

- Cod liver oil (very rich in vitamin A and D).

The above supplement regimen is just the icing on the cake to my diet, and the 2 together (diet plus supplementation) make my nutritional approach. I already get enough macronutrients and micronutrients from my diet, so the daily doses that I use for my supplements are taken into consideration with what I am going to be eating for the day. If I am going to be eating 2 pounds of steak, there is no need for me to take zinc, or if I am going to be ingesting considerable amounts of dairy, I will skip the calcium (or only take a minimal amount).

There are other supplements around that I have used in the past and have helped towards an awesome mane, but these are the ones that I take consistently and have been of long-term benefit to my hair as well as overall heath.

The keys to my nutritional approach

As you have been able to read from the diet that I use for my awesome mane, my diet is high in protein, low in carbohydrates and moderate in fat intake, and it is based around nutrient-dense natural foods. My diet is rich in protein and contains a good source of natural fats; I do not get my fat intake from fast foods, and I instead get my intake from natural foods while emphasising an optimal ratio of omega-3:omega-6 essential fatty acids (1:2 is good for me). I avoid food that has been processed heavily, and I allow myself for infrequent meal treats. Moreover, I use nutritional supplements to complement my diet and not the other way around.

If I were to boil down my nutritional approach to 6 essential points, I would go with the following personal recommendations for an awesome mane:

1) Take in an adequate amount of protein

While the Reference Daily Intake (RDI) for protein for an adult male is easy to achieve (it's about 60 grams), I always take in more and strive to hit 0.8 grams per pound of body weight. That means that if my body weight is 200lbs, I will ingest about 160 grams of protein per day, sometimes even going higher or lower than that. I must note that I engage in heavy strength training, and an increased protein intake is suitable for strength athletes. However, I have experimented with taking lower quantities of protein (including only the established RDI), and I have found not only my training recovery impaired but also the health of my hair (most notably, a weaker tensile strength of the hair strands). From my experiments and findings, 0.8 grams per pound of body weight is my perfect number for hair health.

Remember that protein contains the building blocks for hair, so you certainly don't want to be malnourished in this macronutrient. The RDI is the bare minimum for an adult male, and I have found a higher intake of protein than that of the established RDI to yield stronger hair strands. A daily protein intake of 0.6 grams per pound of body weight is the lowest amount from which I have noticed a positive effect on my hair, whether it was during a period of my life in which I was weightlifting or whether it was during a period in which I didn't lift heavy weights. Likewise, other men who have followed my advice in the past have reported back that 0.6 grams per pound of bodyweight is also their minimal number to grow strong hair strands.

From my experience and findings, a daily protein intake of 0.6 grams per pound of body weight is an optimal one for sedentary individuals who want better hair while a higher daily intake (over 0.8 g/lbs) is better suited for those who engage in any form of frequent weight training. Make sure to consult your doctor first before increasing your protein intake as this nutritional point can only be done if your body is healthy (e.g. healthy kidneys).

2) Increase your fish oil intake

While increasing your intake of fish oil is a great action (i.e. part of the strategy) for optimal hair health, it is not always reasonable to be eating fish every day. First, not every fish has adequate amounts of oils, one needs to eat oily fish such as salmon, sardines or the liver of cod fish. Second, there is a risk of ingesting too much mercury from eating the bigger types of fish too frequently (e.g. shark or swordfish). Mercury is a chemical element that accumulates through the food chain, meaning that the biggest of sea predators will have the highest levels of mercury in their meat.

Fish oil contains an awesome-mane-friendly type of fats: omega-3. Omega-3 is the name for a bunch of essential fatty acids that enhance optimal sebum production and secretion and that most of us males don't ingest enough of. Omega-3 fatty acids are essential for the proper functioning of the body, so lacking in their intake will manifest itself physically. If you are not taking in optimal levels of omega-3s, your hair will be brittle and frizzy, and you will not be maximising your own sebum via the Sebum Coating method.

I have found that 3 grams of omega-3 fatty acids per day is excellent for my awesome mane. While achieving this intake through food alone is doable, supplements in the form of fish-oil gel capsules are extremely convenient. On top of that, the best fish-oil brands ensure the removal of any toxic pollutants that could be found in the extracted oil itself, so, with supplements, you get your optimal intake of fish oil in a convenient manner while avoiding exposure to mercury and other toxic elements.

Lastly, most vegetable oils and fats (especially ones used for cooking) contain too much omega-6 fatty acids and too little omega-3 fatty acids, and it is the balance of your "omega-3:omega-6" intake ratio that matters especially for cardiovascular health and inflammation in the body (male pattern baldness is thought to be partially mediated via chronic inflammation in the scalp). Thus, it is imperative that you get omega-3 fatty acids in your diet so as to balance said omega 3:omega 6 intake ratio. Ideally, you want to have a ratio of 1:2 (or even 1:1), and a typical pro-disease Western diet is 1:15.

3) Vitamin A is king for a healthy scalp

I first experienced the benefits of vitamin A on my scalp while experimenting with fish oil. I had been recording the results of a few trials I had done with fish oil supplements when I decided to give cod liver oil some 8 weeks of trialling. Cod liver oil is a specific type of fish oil that is extremely rich in vitamin A. Most conventional fish oil supplements have trivial amounts of vitamin A whereas cod liver oil not only offers a great source of omega-3 fatty acids but it is also one of nature's best sources of vitamin A (and vitamin D too).

While my notes showed a noticeable benefit from fish oil on how healthy and shiny my curls looked, when I trialled cod liver oil I also noticed a much lower rate of skin flaking (i.e. shedding dead skin cells). During these experiments, I was sporting my mane in a High and Tight Recon on purpose since this hairstyle allowed me to keep the sides and back of my head shaved and thus be able to document any changes in scalp health.

With cod liver oil, I noticed a scalp benefit that I didn't notice with fish oil. I was shaving my scalp every 2 days, and every time that I would shave my hair during the cod liver oil trial, the shaved scalp would not become irritated and red. On the other hand, every time that I shaved my scalp when I was taking fish oil alone, I would experience mild irritation from the razor, and the skin would turn a light red for a few hours. Once I finished the trial with cod liver oil, I decided to resume the use of fish oil, but I also started taking vitamin A at a dose equating the dose ingested in the cod liver oil trial (through the cod liver oil itself), and, lo and behold, I experienced the same anti-irritation and skin-smoothing benefit of cold liver oil! Vitamin A has been known for decades to be nature's skin moisturiser and is a vitamin that is highly underrated.

Bear in mind that the scalp contains the thriving part of your hair; the scalp contains the follicles that continuously produce new hair material. A healthy scalp contains, by default, healthy hair follicles, which in turn equates healthy hair strands (i.e. glossier and stronger); this is why your hair care strategy must target the hair follicles too, not just the hair strands. Vitamin A is one of the best vitamins to use to notice a boost in hair quality starting from the very root (pun intended).

If you want to use cod liver oil, be aware that it tastes even worse than plain fish oil, so you are better off buying gel caps instead of the liquid. Also, be aware that cod liver oil is very rich in vitamin D, and you should consult your doctor prior to using cod liver oil as your own skin makes vitamin D when exposed to sunlight, hence using cod liver oil may push your vitamin D levels to higher than desired for optimal health. Furthermore, fish oil (including cod liver oil) can anticoagulate your blood when taken in very high doses or if taken when anticoagulation medication is being used (e.g. warfarin).

If you choose not to use cod liver oil, make sure that you are ingesting optimal amounts of other vitamin A-rich sources such as eggs, beef liver and dairy. Lastly, if you go down the supplement route, buy vitamin A in the form of retinol and not beta-carotene as the former is much stronger than the latter.

4) Whole eggs are superfoods

I view whole eggs as superfoods. They are choked with essential vitamins and minerals, and they even contain some omega-3 fatty acids. Eggs are an excellent source of protein and sulphur, the latter being a mineral associated with stronger hair strands. Moreover, eggs can be a staple food for those who don't eat meat since many of the essential micronutrients in meat are also found in eggs.

With eggs, I have noticed a special benefit in terms of the strength of my hair. Since eggs are nature's multivitamin, my hair has looked great every time that my egg intake was higher than what most men ingest (4+ whole eggs per day). Call me, perhaps, a good responder to eggs, but I have always found my hair and body strength to be at its peak when I was eating eggs in abundance.

Scientists have found out in the laboratory that most nutrients are best absorbed and best utilised when they are ingested as they are found in nature. Calcium is a perfect example, the fat naturally found in milk enhances the absorption of calcium, which makes milk a superior source of calcium than calcium supplements alone. Thus, I would not be surprised if, with eggs, the synergies of all the nutrients in the yolk and the albumen yielded a superior form of hair-optimising nutrients such as protein, fatty acids, sulphur and vitamin A.

Again, if you are going to emulate my high consumption of eggs, consult a doctor first because you may end up negatively affecting your cholesterol levels.

5) Berries and fruits for those antioxidants

Not only are fruits nature's tasty desserts but many fruits are also great sources of antioxidants, vitamins and nutrients that are not found anywhere else in nature. I am a huge fan of berries in their culinary (not botanical) definition: blueberries, strawberries, raspberries and redberries are my favourites although, if I had to pick one, I'd go with blueberries because they are a packed with huge amounts of antioxidants. Blueberries are tasty, can be used to make smoothies and milk shakes, can be sprinkled on pretty much anything, and they have an excellent nutrient profile.

While the tangible hair benefit from eating berries hasn't been as pronounced as the hair benefit from ingesting fish oil and vitamin A, I have certainly found a great hair benefit from complementing my diet with extra vitamin C, a vitamin found in vast amounts in all berries. Many times, it is the lack of certain nutrients in one's diet that leads to tangible and noticeable negative effects on one's hair, and, with blueberries in my diet, I do know for sure that my vitamin C intake is more than satisfied.

As I've mentioned in the previous point, nutrients are best utilised by the body as they are found in nature, so the vitamin C found in berries is highly useful and efficiently absorbed for our hair-optimising purposes. Thus, strive to often ingest fruits and especially berries, for you will be building with these the foundation to a nutritional approach that is excellent in its micronutrient intake.

6) Use of nutritional supplements as a complement to your diet

Also known as food supplements or dietary supplements, nutritional supplements do absolutely have a place in one's nutritional approach. You cannot always ensure that you are getting the highest amounts of nutrients from the foods you eat, so nutritional supplements allow you to bulletproof your diet and overall nutrition. The problem is that many men think of nutritional supplements as magic pills that, when taken in excess, will lead to whatever it is that the supplement's manufacturer claims. Not only is thinking of nutritional supplements as magic pills a waste of your time but their excessive intake may also prove dangerous or counterproductive. To use nutritional supplements the right way, you should research them first and use them to complement your diet so as to create an optimal nutritional approach.

The following nutritional supplements are of great use exclusively for your awesome mane:

- Zinc (taken with copper in a 10:1 ratio).

- Vitamin A, D and E (taken separately or together and preferably with a meal).

- The whole spectrum of the B vitamins, especially biotin (vitamin B7).

- Vitamin C with citrus flavonoids.

- Iodine as a supplement alone or in the form of iodised salt or kelp.

- Fish oil or cod liver oil.

- Methylsulfonylmethane (MSM).

- A multivitamin with 100% of the RDI for all vitamins and minerals.

- Whey protein if you find that you cannot meet your optimal intake of protein via food alone.

All of the above when taken as nutritional supplements and when added to an optimal diet will lead to better hair. Any time that you want to introduce a supplement into your nutritional approach, make sure that you research it thoroughly and that you consult your doctor before; some nutritional supplements may actually lead to micronutrient deficiencies or may accumulate beyond safe levels, so tread carefully. My advice is to obtain 100% of the RDI for all vitamins and minerals via supplementation so that you bulletproof your nutritional approach without risking toxic levels of micronutrients.

My personal experience

As I was on the path to achieving my awesome mane, I learnt that even the best of manes will have to face daily issues. I remember one day sitting at my desk with a blank paper in front me and writing down all the problems that I was facing back then with my curls as I tried to look at the bigger picture. I narrowed down all my hair dramas to 3 universal factors that were also true for the rest of the curly men I knew: dry hair, tangled hair and hair loss. Fortunately, I was not hit by hair loss at the time although I was well aware that this is an issue that the majority of men, including yours truly, have to face at one time or another.

Through the years, I have learnt that being proactive is the best way to approach the care of one's mane. This is because by being proactive, you get to avoid the time-consuming reactive measures, and you also get to learn about your hair with such a preventive approach. Sure, some of the proactive measures are a bit annoying, but most of them can become an easy habit. For example, I always use an extra amount of leave-in conditioner by default when it is windy outside; I have learnt that, on windy days, I can leave my house with an awesome mane, only to find that 15 minutes later I have a dead rat on top of my head. The convertible story was the straw that broke the camel's back, and it taught me that, with curly hair, there's no overdoing it in terms of hair care.

To this day, my awesome mane still becomes dry if I don't keep up with my hair grooming, still tangles like crazy if I rub my head on the pillow with my untied medium-length curls, and I still lose some hair strands here and there from unintentionally pulling my hair as I tie my hair when it is long. For most of the time, however, my awesome mane is as healthy as it needs to be.

Just like any other modern male, I too have gone through very stressful periods in my life, which is why earlier on I felt the need to briefly address a problem that is endemic in our fast-moving society. Having lived in 5 countries, I have at times been alone while I had to prioritise my professional career over my personal life, and I can certainly relate to those men who have to pile a lot of responsibilities on their shoulders or have to be away from their loved ones for considerable amounts of time.

In terms of the nutritional approach to my awesome mane, well, you have read it straight from the horse's mouth. I have used this approach for years, and it is the best that I can do for the health of my hair. Doing the Sebum Coating method with this nutritional approach is extremely easy as I find my curls to be effortlessly sebuminised without me having to work my fingers hard on the locks. Likewise, this nutritional approach is the best that I can do for my overall health too, so I am very happy using it with my modern lifestyle and now putting it into this book for you to obtain some nutritional inspiration and ideas for your curls and overall health.

5) Achieving The Physical Part: Putting Your Mane Together

"Even a mistake may turn out to be the one thing necessary to a worthwhile achievement"

Henry Ford

This chapter covers the extra stuff that you can do to enhance your head of curls, and it consolidates everything that has been covered in the previous chapters so as to put together the physical part of your awesome mane. Of course, your awesome mane includes an important mental part that will be covered in the next chapter, but, by the end of this chapter, you will have learnt all the hair-specific aspects and elements relating to the physical part of your awesome mane.

To be able to put your mane together, you will be confident in your hair grooming as you will have learnt all there is to it in the third chapter "Hair Grooming: Get Those Curls Looking Great" and you will also be acquainted with your hair care and your curly hair 101 from having previously read the chapters "Hair Care: Looking After Your Healthy Awesome Mane" and "Curly Hair 101: Know Your Waves, Coils Or Kinks". You will not be spinning your wheels any more with your hair because you have fully grasped the notion of knowing that which inhabits your head, and you are now ready to approach its daily grooming in a methodical manner while ensuring its daily hair care over the long term. Indeed, it is the proper grooming and caring of your curly hair that creates the foundation of your awesome mane, and the enhancements that are to be covered in this chapter are what will give the shape and form to said awesome mane.

So, once you have your hair grooming and hair care to a T and your awesome mane is looking the part, it is time to consider a suiting hairstyle, to hit the barber for the right trim or haircut, and to even consider using hair accessories; it will be the integration of all these final elements into your awesome mane foundation that will put the physical part together.

Hairstyles for your awesome mane

When it comes to hairstyles, we curly dudes don't have it easy. What is feasible for a Type V is not feasible for a Type I and vice versa. Unlike straight haired dudes, we can't just open a magazine and choose any of the hairstyles that we see, our manes are not made that way. Through the years, I have found the majority of curly dudes to be reluctant and resistant to trying any hairstyles on their curls simply because their hair grooming and caring routine was subpar (if it actually existed). As a curly haired dude, it is once you get your hair grooming and hair care sorted that the rest, including hairstyles, will flow naturally.

It is very important to be realistic about what hairstyles can and cannot be done on your awesome mane. Whatever your curl type may be, you have styling options available, so don't worry about the flashy hairstyles that you see in magazines and that make you feel bad about your curls because you can't copy those uber/trendy/fabulous (insert hip word) hairstyles. You are already sporting an awesome mane, and it has become a part of your own self: this is what truly matters and what will elevate your confidence in yourself and have you finally proud and happy with that which flourishes atop your head.

Haircut vs. Hairstyle

Before we go into the hairstyles that I recommend for each curl type, it is imperative that you are aware of the difference between a haircut and a hairstyle, for these terms tend to be confused and misinterpreted by many guys.

As it goes, to rock a certain hairstyle you first need the proper haircut. Many of us, myself included, have made the mistake of using both terms interchangeably despite each conveying something different. Sure, they both relate to hair, but a "haircut" involves cutting while a "hairstyle" involves styling. I want you to be sure of the meaning of each because, for your awesome mane efforts, you will sooner or later get a haircut and try a hairstyle.

Haircut

A haircut refers to the specific act of trimming or cutting the hair so that it is given a shape. It is done in the moment and can be regarded as part of a routine to cut the length of the hair every so often, or it can be done with a specific cosmetic goal in mind (e.g. give the hair a certain shape for a hairstyle you have in mind). A haircut is commonly done with scissors (aka shears) and/or a hair clipper. An example of a haircut is a buzz cut: cropping the hair to a very short length all around the head and performed with a hair clipper.

Hairstyle

This refers to the modification and manipulation of the hair without cutting it so that it looks in a certain form or shape. Having said that, a hairstyle can also be regarded as the final hair shape obtained after a haircut as the shape obtained is the one desired to be worn daily until the next haircut. With men, a hairstyle is most commonly thought of in the long term; that is, a hairstyle would be worn for weeks or months at a time according to the preference of the individual although a hairstyle can also be worn for a single or specific occasion. Some common hairstyles for curly dudes include the Afro (Type III-V) or the Side Swept (Type I-II).

As it relates to your awesome mane, you go to the barber to get a haircut and you give yourself a hairstyle every morning after you get out of the shower to implement the third stage of your hair grooming routine. You can get a haircut done to specifically sport a hairstyle, or you can simply go for a haircut every number of weeks to keep your hair at a certain length. Likewise, you can also give yourself a haircut instead of going to the barber although I recommend you to only do this if you truly master the art of cutting hair and, even then, limit it to giving yourself small trims as you run the risk of ruining your awesome mane in an instant (I speak from experience!).

Hairstyles are typically done in the bathroom as part of your daily hair grooming after you are done with the conditioning stage and approach the styling stage. However, you can give yourself a hairstyle under other scenarios not requiring the previous two stages of the hair grooming routine; all you have to bear in mind is to always dampen your hair prior to styling it: never give yourself a hairstyle on non-damp hair as that is a recipe for disaster, though you can retouch the hairstyle without having to dampen your hair again.

Hairstyles for curl types

It is imperative for you to know that not all hairstyles will be suitable for your awesome mane. I am not here to sell you dreams; that is not my job. Unless you love spending much of your free time in hair salons having your hair retouched while drinking tea and discussing the latest Hollywood gossip with your hairstylist, you should then stick to those hairstyles that suit your curl type. Absolutely every curl type can be styled with cool and suitable hairstyles; you just need to know which ones are feasible for your type of curly hair.

I recommend you to go for the simpler and more convenient hairstyles; basically, go for those hairstyles that are easy to stay with and that you can give yourself in a moment. Elaborate hairstyles look great in magazines and photo shoots, but they are not convenient for modern curly men because they involve great investments in time and effort, not to mention money as you will have to be frequently visiting the hair salon to keep the chosen hairstyle looking neat. Of course, for once-in-a-while occasions, feel free to go nuts with elaborate hairstyles if that's what you want, but do not make them a daily thing because an awesome mane has a convenience factor that is shot down with elaborate hairstyles.

While there is a range to choose from in terms of awesome-mane-friendly hairstyles, I advise you to first consider the beautifully-simple Shake & Go hairstyle as a starting point to experimenting with hairstyles on your awesome mane.

The Shake & Go hairstyle is done by making your hair damp (e.g. after a shower), coating the curls with whichever hairstyling agent you decide to go with and then shaking your head briefly to allow the curls to sit on top of your head freely. The curls will just sit there, showing their natural form and looking awesome, provided that you have already mastered your hair grooming routine and hair care strategy. The Shake & Go is a favourite hairstyle of mine, and it works well with all curl types especially when they are at medium lengths.

The cool thing about starting with the Shake & Go hairstyle before venturing into the rest of hairstyles available is that you will get to know how your curls react, adapt and express with the hairstyling agent you use. If you try the Shake & Go hairstyle for a week, you will be able to learn how your hair reacts without being manipulated and you'll familiarise yourself with the Damp vs. Dry effect, with all of this then paving the way for optimally choosing further hairstyles. Moreover, the Shake & Go hairstyle is suitable for all types of curls and will never let you down during those times when you just can't be bothered to choose a hairstyle for the day and want something fast and aesthetic.

What follows are my recommended hairstyles for each curl type and hair length. By all means, they are not the only ones available for each curl type, and you can try the hairstyles that I recommend for the curl types that precede and follow your particular curl type (e.g. if you have Type III curls, you can try the hairstyles for Type II or Type IV curls). The recommended hairstyles that you will find below for your specific curl type will, however, suit you optimally.

Type I

Type I curls, colloquially known as wavy, are the closest of all curl types to straight hair, and many of the short-length hairstyles available to straight haired dudes are also applicable to Type I curly haired guys. If you have Type I short curls, you can try any of the hairstyles you may see done on short straight hair. You won't have much of an issue with your hair looking different between damp and dry states, so you can do most hairstyles knowing that your hair will still look the same at the end of the day as it did at the start of the day when it was styled. Wax, pomades, hair gel and mousse are the hairstyling agents that will work great for styling your awesome mane.

- Spikes (short length)

This hairstyle is very popular among males, and it revolves around lifting one's hair to create the illusion of spikes. Use hair gel to lift your curls up, and, once you have lifted them all, use your fingers to go lock by lock to further define their spike shape, rapidly running the fingers from mid-length to the tip so as to ensure that all locks are coated with hair gel. You can do all the hair on your head or only do the spikes on the top of your head.

A perfect example of the Spikes hairstyle is Taylor Lautner's hair from The Twilight Saga films.

- The Side Fringe (medium length)

With this hairstyle, you will part your hair from either the left or right temple. You will have the front of your hair covering your forehead (i.e. fringe) and styled in your desired direction. You choose how much you want the fringe to cover your forehead. Use a wide-tooth comb and run it smoothly through the locks as you part them to the side and set the fringe on your forehead. Try to use the smallest amount of your chosen hairstyling agent on the fringe so as to avoid getting the product on your forehead; your fringe will hold up in place with little product.

The Side Fringe is best exemplified in the movie <u>17 Again</u> by Zac Efron.

- <u>The Shoulder Length (long length)</u>

This hairstyle involves growing your mane to reach the shoulders or base of the neck. It requires the hair to be trimmed in layers so that all of it reaches the shoulders and doesn't exceed this length mark. For your curl type, the hair at the very top of your head will require an extended length of about 15 inches to reach the shoulders whereas the hair at the nape will only need about 6 inches of extended length, hence the need to trim the hair in layers as it grows.

You are best growing the Shoulder Length hairstyle by first getting a haircut that has all your hair at an even length all around your head so that you start growing your curls from the same length. Then, trim the hair as each segment of the scalp reaches the shoulders.

The Shoulder Length is perfectly illustrated by Antonio Banderas in the movie <u>Desperado</u>.

Type II

Since this curl type mostly forms waves instead of coils, many of the hairstyle recommendations on Type I do also apply to Type II. However, because the curls formed in Type II are a bit tighter than Type I, one should pay special attention to the Damp vs. Dry (DvD) effect. If you have medium or long Type II curly hair, make sure that you use some hair gel along with your leave-in conditioner to ensure that your mane doesn't surprise you with the DvD effect. Pomade, hair gel, hair mousse and wax (use wax only at short and medium lengths) are your best products to use; the leave-in conditioner is used as a hairstyling foundation (i.e. applied first), and it starts to become a necessity at medium lengths.

- <u>The Caesar Cut (short length)</u>

This is a short-length hairstyle that involves having your back and sides of the head cropped with a hair clipper (preferably done as a taper) while leaving the top trimmed evenly with any length between 0.5 to 1 inches. You style the hair on the top of your head in a forward direction, starting from the crown area and ending at the forehead's hairline as you leave a short vertical fringe laying on the forehead. Use a wide-tooth comb to style the hair forward and your fingers to further style the short fringe.

An awesome mane example of the Caesar Cut is that of George Clooney in the 1996 movie <u>From Dusk Till Dawn</u>.

- The Side Swept (medium length)

This is a medium-length hairstyle in which you have your sides and back trimmed up to 1 inch while leaving the top between 2-4 inches. All the hair on the top is parted (swept) to one side, and the line of division for the part is drawn starting at either the left or right temple of your head. Unlike the Side Fringe hairstyle, which also shares the side parting at the temple, there is no fringe here: all of the hair on the top of the head is parted to the side so that the newly-swept hair remains perpendicular or at an angle to the parted line created.

A dude who wears the Side Swept with style and class is Billy Zane in the movie <u>Titanic</u>.

- The Jim Morrison (long length)

The Jim Morrison is a hairstyle named after the rock star himself, Jim Morrison. To achieve this hairstyle, you need 6 inches of hair all around your head. To style a Jim Morrison, use hair mousse to lift your hair up so that it ends up looking like a helmet. Use your fingers to lift the hair up, aiming to create a visual helmet-like effect. If you use a leave-in conditioner normally as your hairstyling foundation, it is best that for this particular hairstyle you either use a smaller-than-usual amount or skip the leave-in altogether to style your mane in a Jim Morrison because the leave-in will weight down your curls. While the Jim Morrison is not a fully puffing-out hairstyle, it certainly requires a messy volume that defies gravity somewhat.

With the Jim Morrison hairstyle, you want to elongate the lifting-up motion of your fingers and solely use hair mousse as a hairstyling agent so that the curls can defy gravity. You can also use a hair dryer to enhance the puffing out of the hair.

Jim Morrison in any of the covers for <u>The Best Of</u> albums of The Doors will serve to illustrate this wild hairstyle.

Type III

Type III curls will have a tendency to defy gravity until they reach at least 8 inches in visible length, and they will puff out when shorter. Because Type III curls are formed as coils rather than waves, you want to use plenty of leave-in conditioner and avoid sweeping or excessively slicking your hair. The Damp vs. Dry effect is noticeable with Type III curly hair so watch out for it: your hair will not look the same when it dries as it did when it was damp and styled! Use a leave-in conditioner at all times, either as a standalone hairstyling agent or as a foundation to other agents; you can also use hair gel, hair mousse, pomade, styling creams and hair spray. Avoid hair wax except for short-length curls and only use it in small amounts.

- The Faux Hawk (short length)

This hairstyle is a trendy one for those Type III curly males. It revolves around styling the hair on the top of the head towards the middle so as to form a crest running from the centre of the forehead's hairline to the crown area. You will need your sides and back tapered to a #2 with a hair clipper, and the top should be anywhere from 0.5 to 2 inches in height (i.e. visible length). The Faux Hawk is a modern alternative to the extreme Mohawk hairstyle and suits short Type III curls greatly. Use your fingers to define the crest and use either your fingers or a wide-tooth comb to direct the hair on the top of the head towards the middle so as to form the crest. The crest can be as wide as you want it to be although 0.5-inches wide all across the crest is a good width to aim for.

A great example of the Faux Hawk hairstyle is that of Cristiano Ronaldo playing for Real Madrid in the 2010-2011 Spanish soccer league.

- The Jewfro (medium length)

The Jewfro is a popular hairstyle for Type III curly men. The name itself comes from the popularity of this hairstyle among males of Jewish heritage, for whom curly hair is a common trait. It is similar in goal to the common Afro hairstyle in that the hair is allowed to puff out and look voluminous. You will need the same length all around your head (preferably 3-5 inches), and you will use hair mousse to lift the hair up when it is damp. Run your fingers coated with hair mousse from mid-length to the tips so that the whole length gets coated with hair mousse, and emphasise the lifting up and puffing out of your curls.

The good thing about hair mousse is that it is easy to remove and hardly leaves any residue, so it is OK if some hair mousse unintentionally coats the base of the hair strands when you are styling your Jewfro. Moreover, while the Jewfro and the Jim Morrison hairstyles share a puffing-out emphasis, you should use some leave-in conditioner for the Jewfro as a foundation prior to applying the hair mousse. You can blow-dry the Jewfro too, but don't go overboard and do leave some dampness on the hair.

Many Type III curly men make the mistake of allowing their hair to become dry and frizzy, which then leads to their curly hair naturally taking the form of a pseudo Jewfro. The thing is, we want an awesome mane, not a frizzy dead rat; hence, the Jewfro should not be the result of allowing the curls to become dry but the result of having a mane that is moisturised and styled accordingly and which looks awesome regardless of the hairstyle. I grow quite the Jewfro myself, and I can tell you that the difference between a dry Jewfro and a moisturised Jewfro is like day and night (not to mention that women love an awesome Jewfro mane as it really flaunts your curls).

An example of a male with an awesome Jewfro is Justin Guarini, a popular American singer who has sported this hairstyle for most of his career since 2002.

- The Hanging Locks (long length)

The Hanging Locks hairstyle is perfect for Type III long curls because it doesn't take a huge amount of time for this curl type to hang down (as opposed to the tight curl types), and the hanging down can be enhanced with the use of hairstyling agents that add weight to the hair strands. With the Hanging Locks hairstyle, you will need 10 inches of extended hair length on the top, and the sides and back should be 8 inches, which will give a very full appearance to your mane.

For the Hanging Locks hairstyle, I recommend you to use a styling cream so as to ensure that the locks hang down, for, at the aforementioned stipulated lengths, Type III curly hair tends not to hang down fully without hair products. Coat your curls with leave-in conditioner first, then add the styling cream. Once the hair is coated with these 2 hairstyling agents, shake your curls and let them hang down freely without parting them to the side. Slick back any locks hanging on your face but don't manipulate the rest of the hair.

A perfect male example of this hairstyle is David Bisbal in the cover of his 2004 album Buleria.

Type IV

This curl type thrives best when not manipulated. If you are the proud owner of Type IV curly hair, do not try to sweep it or dominate it with hairstyles. Type IV is a step up from Type III in terms of volume, and your best approach is to embrace the natural volume yielded by your curls, hence it is with Type IV curly hair that the Shake & Go hairstyle is of greatest use. In this curl type, the curls are very tight and formed as coils, so the Damp vs. Dry effect is very noticeable once the curls reach a medium length; thus, you should not try to fight your hair and instead embrace its voluminous and coiling nature.

A leave-in conditioner is a must, and natural oils and butters are great add-ons for your styling stage. Hair gels, pomades and styling creams are also great options though try to emphasise the use of a leave-in conditioner as the foundation for your styling and then add the rest of your chosen hairstyling agents, paying particular attention to not getting any of them on your scalp.

• The High and Tight (short length)

The High and Tight is a great hairstyle for those with Type IV curls who want to sport a low-maintenance, good-looking hairstyle. With the High and Tight, you will crop the back and sides of your scalp to a #2 while the top is left anywhere from a #4 to a trimmed length of up to 1 inch. You can go lower than a #2 with the guard length for the sides and back, but do a #2 first, then leave 2-3 weeks before you crop the hair shorter to make sure that your scalp gets tanned naturally to the same tone as your face, otherwise you will have a disturbing skin tone discrepancy between your face and the sides and back of your head. The top of your head can either be styled with your fingers or styled with a wide-tooth comb.

A great example of a High and Tight is that of Shemar Moore in the TV show Criminal Minds.

- The Shake & Go (medium length)

Because Type IV curls tend to have very defined curls, the Shake & Go hairstyle is perfect to flaunt that awesome mane of yours. Get your curls to an even medium length (preferably 4-5 inches) all around your head; to style, simply coat your damp Type IV curls with a leave-in conditioner and your other chosen hairstyling agents, then shake your head, and you are ready to go. Since you will have an awesome mane already, your curls will be allowed to express themselves while looking great as you will have developed the habits needed to have great-looking curly hair. For the Shake & Go hairstyle, you can finish off the styling stage by adding a fingertip amount of coconut butter or any other natural oil or butter to the tip of your curls for an extra hair-conditioning layer.

The Shake & Go is very similar in concept to the Hanging Locks hairstyle for Type III curly men, only that, with the Shake & Go hairstyle as done on Type IV medium-length curls, your hair will not hang down and will instead defy gravity.

Corbin Bleu, in the TV movie High School Musical, is a great male illustration of the Shake & Go hairstyle.

- The Beyond Shoulder Length (long length)

This hairstyle requires you to grow your awesome mane beyond shoulder length. A good length to aim for is chest length because at this length your locks will be hanging down while expressing great volume: a true lion's mane! If you are growing from a short length, this hairstyle will take you +5 years to achieve, but it is a great hairstyle if you want to really sport an impressive head of curls. What's more is that since you will be growing your curls already as an awesome mane, your hair will be looking great throughout the entire journey that it takes you to have your hair reaching its final length.

For the Beyond Shoulder Length hairstyle, it is best that you grow your mane starting from an even length all around your head. Moreover, you should not go for trims until you achieve the final length desired (only go for trims if you have damaged the tips of the hair). It is imperative to keep your hair free of tangles with this hairstyle as you can get some vicious knots and tangles appearing very fast, so use a leave-in conditioner every day and a normal conditioner on just about all days too.

NFL player Troy Polamalu of the Pittsburgh Steelers is the perfect example of what Type IV curly hair grown beyond shoulder length can look like.

Type V

With Type V curly hair (i.e. kinks), the superbly-tight curls will not hang down unless they are severely weighted down, which means that if you have this curl type, you must embrace your ability to grow a lot of gravity-defying volume. If you desire a long length for your awesome mane, you can either continue with an Afro hairstyle or use braids or dreadlocks to weight the hair down. I have found that many guys with Type V curls tend to prefer to crop their heads very short and forget about their hair, but, if you have this curl type, I can assure you that you can do many things with your hair once you have established your awesome mane foundation. Your optimal hairstyling agents to use are: leave-in conditioners, natural oils and butters, and styling creams.

- The Crew Cut (short length)

This hairstyle is great for short-length Type V curls as it is convenient and can be customised as per one's taste. The top is cropped very short and tapered from the crown towards the front so that the front has a little bit more length than the crown. The sides and back are kept even shorter, from a #1 to a #2, and done in a taper too. This hairstyle is similar to the High and Tight, only that the length differences between the top and the sides and back are much smaller and less noticeable. Another cool thing of this hairstyle is that you can customise it with lines and even patches of shaved hair, making elaborate designs as the length of the hairstyle itself is very short anyway, which allows for creative dents in the hair (I recommend you to have the barber do it, not do it yourself).

A great example of how good a Crew Cut hairstyle can look on a Type V curly male is the hair of United State's President Barack Obama in his earlier political career as a senator.

- The Afro (medium length)

This hairstyle is the everest of mane awesomeness for Type V curly dudes. If your curls are Type V, the Afro hairstyle is a great way to acknowledge your mane, and this hairstyle always looks great when it is taken care of. Most commonly a medium-length hairstyle, your Afro should have an even length all around your head, with the chosen even length for your curls ranging from 2 to 6 inches. It is imperative for you to keep your Afro moisturised daily with plenty of leave-in conditioner and by coating the tips with natural oils and butters because the main problem with not achieving mane awesomeness with the Afro hairstyle is failing to keep the kinks moisturised.

The Afro hairstyle is greatly illustrated by Lenny Kravitz any time that he is not sporting dreadlocks or a Buzz Cut (he seems to prefer the Afro for his medium-length hairstyle).

- Braids (long length)

Braids are a favourite for men with long Type V curls. Due to the tightness of the kinks, this curl type has a tendency to defy gravity even at very long lengths. Instead, braids pair up the long curly locks, allowing them to be weighted down and thus hang down. A good way to approach the braided hairstyle is to transition from an Afro to braids: once your Afro reaches a good-enough long length that you are happy with (e.g. 10 inches), then braid your mane. It should be noted, however, that the braiding process and braids themselves put a lot of tension on the hair follicles, and this hairstyle can cause some unneeded hair loss if the hair is braided too tight, so you certainly want to use someone who knows how to braid hair if you decide to have your awesome mane braided.

Rapper Snoop Dogg is an awesome male example of how to rock braids as a Type V curly male.

How to choose the right barber

Many times, we curly dudes underestimate the benefit of having a good barber or hairdresser. Indeed, to be able to rock an awesome mane, you also need to be in the hands of a good hair professional. Not all barbers and hairdressers are created equal, and you want to choose one who has experience with your curl type (or at least with curly hair) and who is also a good listener.

How many times have you stepped inside a barbershop or hair salon to get a haircut and left with something completely different to what you wanted? How many times did you trust the barber to do what he felt was right, only to find that what he thought was right differed vastly from what you thought was right? If you are like me, your experiences with barbers and hairdressers are more on the bad side than on the good side, and you try to avoid them unless necessary.

An awesome mane relies on you doing everything right, but when the time comes for a good haircut (and it will come), you can either do it yourself or have someone else doing it for you. And while I am one who thinks that for things to go your way, you need to be the one doing them; a good haircut is best relied on a hair professional. By all means, have a go at cutting your own hair and learn how to give yourself frequent trims, but I recommend you to go to a barber or hairdresser whenever you need a good haircut.

Once you achieve your awesome mane, you will learn to appreciate your curls, and your first time stepping inside a barber or hair salon with your awesome mane will give you butterflies in the stomach. Due to your newly-found appreciation for your hair, you will not be very receptive to someone else touching and manipulating your hair, so you must know how to choose the right professional for your haircut. I have walked out of a barbershop after being there for 5 minutes and seeing the guy who went before me getting a horrible haircut by a hairdresser who thought a "hip" haircut consisted of leaving lumps of hair on each side of the head while buzzing the top. The guy getting the haircut didn't look like he was enjoying having the hairdresser (or "hairkiller" as it looked) freestyling a haircut on his head, and I was pretty much terrified of having that hairdresser dude within 10 feet of my head.

To ensure choosing the best barber or hairdresser right from the very beginning and getting the most out of him/her, follow these points:

- Be 100% sure of what haircut you want. Practise describing what haircut you want to a friend or family member: if they can understand what you want done, a hair professional will have no problems catching your 100% drift.

- Take pictures with you to the barber. Take magazines, printed pictures, newspaper clippings or whatever illustrations needed to show him what it is that you want done.

- A good barber/hairdresser should know how to cut hair when dry. Curly hair should be cut dry most of the time because, if it is cut when wet or damp, it is difficult to assess how the haircut will look when the hair dries due to the Damp vs. Dry effect. Ask him if he is familiarised with cutting hair dry.

- Be realistic, not all haircuts will suit you. While George Clooney may look awesome with a Caesar Cut, you may not fare just as well because you don't have his facial structure. Ideally, you want to have 3 haircuts in mind and discuss with the barber which one of the 3 would suit you best. Barbers and hairdressers have seen and worked on all sort of faces and hair, so they will be able to advise you on how each haircut will suit you.

- Remember, a good barber/hairdresser always listens to you. You should spend about 5 minutes in the beginning talking about what you want done, and you should be asking him for his opinion, feedback, and any alternatives he has to what you have proposed. Don't worry about being overly detailed and spend as much time as needed to make sure that you both are on the same page. It only takes him 2 seconds to chop by mistake 1 inch from a hair lock of yours, yet it will take you at least 2 months to grow back that lost hair length. Go out of your way to be as precise and detailed as possible so that he/she can then deliver a good job.

- Be aware at all times that a haircut is different from a hairstyle, and sometimes even barbers get themselves confused with these 2 terms. A haircut can be done in minutes, but a hairstyle will require you to style your hair day in and day out. Are you sure you want to get a specific haircut that only allows you to style your hair in a particular hairstyle every day for the next 2 months? If you want to be flexible with hairstyles, choose a haircut that will allow you to choose from several hairstyles in any given day and that will not limit you to just one.

- For us dudes, barbers tend to be a better option than hairdressers when it comes to an awesome mane. Barbers are used to cutting hair for males who want good hair but also want convenient hair. Hairdressers (and hairstylists), on the other hand, tend to be experienced in giving haircuts that look good in the given moment but are a pain in the derriere to style every day. Overall, I find barbers to be more suited for awesome

(follows from previous page)

manes than hairdressers, but there are some pretty good hairdressers out there too. Research him/her fully before making your decision, and do not hesitate to visit him and have a chat with him or his assistants before making a decision.

- Try to find a barber/hairdresser who has plenty of experience with curly hair and especially with your curl type. Curly hair is different to cut than straight hair, and there are bits and pieces that a barber/hairdresser needs to master to be able to provide a good haircut to a curly haired male. Ask him how much experience he has with curly hair and with your specific curl type.

- Female barbers/hairdressers are just as capable as males in delivering a great haircut. The only thing different is that a male barber will be obviously more aware of your needs as a man. All other things equal, I normally go for a male barber because I know that I can relate to him in terms of sporting a masculine haircut. Likewise, it totally kills my mood to have to be waiting my turn in a hair salon full of old women with foil covering their hair and reading the latest issue of Cosmopolitan. Horses for courses though, and, as I say, both genders are equally capable of delivering a great haircut and service.

- Don't go by price. My best haircut was done in Alabama by a barber who charged me $6. My worst haircut was one I had in London by a hairdresser who charged me $35 for a fade and scissor-trimmed top (I was new in the city and desperate for a haircut). Actually, let me take that back: my best haircut ever was when I was 21 and my friends and I were at a house party doing tequila contests. I beat one of my friends, so I, in a drunken stupor, asked him to cut my hair in front of everyone in the house. He was even more drunk than I was and had his right hand in a sling, yet he miraculously got to performing on my scalp an awesome High and Tight that looked out of this world. We are talking about cutting hair here, not performing brain surgery, so there's no need to break the bank to get a great and convenient haircut.

- Arrive at the hair salon some 15 minutes before scheduled so that you can see how your chosen hair professional performs his job with someone else (why be the guinea pig when you can have someone else be experimented on?). See how much attention the barber/hairdresser pays to what he is doing and if he is detailed enough. Try to hear if he chats while performing the haircut. I recommend you to never choose a barber/hairdresser who doesn't look like he is paying much attention to the haircut or talks too much while doing his job. While I understand that a barber or a hairdresser might have to be on his feet cutting hair for 10+ hours, it is a reality that one cannot do 2 things perfectly at the same time. Moreover, if he is doing all the talking, it means he is not doing the listening (to you).

135

- Do not be afraid to walk out of the barbershop/hair salon if you are not 100% sure of the hairdresser's ability to deliver a professional service. You would not be the first one to walk out on a hairdresser, and you would not be the last one either. Remember, you now have an awesome mane, not a dead rat that can be abused and cut like a rag. Be aware though that you may still be liable for paying the unperformed service, especially if you made an appointment.

- Lastly, build a relationship with your barber or hairdresser. This is because you want him to know your hair and your circumstances, which will allow him to offer you the best service possible. Strive to find someone who fits the profile shaped by the above points: good listener, professional and has experience with curly hair. Once you find him or her, do not let him go because a good barber/hairdresser is hard to find for a second time!

Hair accessories to enhance your awesome mane

Men have used hair accessories for centuries, either as ornaments for their manes to showcase their social status or as tools to keep their hair fixed when engaging in battle or physical activity. The popularity of hair accessories faded as shorter hairstyles became more popular at the turn of the 20th century, but hair accessories have made a comeback in the last decade as urban men have started to enhance their image in the most creative of manners.

The following are the hair accessories that I recommend for your awesome mane:

- Headbands

- Hair bands

- Bobby pins

- Do-rags

- Hair picks

The above 5 hair accessories serve a tangible purpose while blending in nicely with your curly hair, and they are the ones that I recommend if you want to enhance your awesome mane.

I will not deny it; the correct use of hair accessories is a bit tricky for us men. You must choose them wisely as it is very easy to ruin your awesome mane; thus, when in doubt, do not wear them. You should bear in mind the following (on the next page) when deciding to wear any hair accessory:

- Discretion: the hair accessory is there to enhance your mane, not to take away from it. Never wear a hair accessory just because you want to show off your latest acquisition. Remember, your awesome mane is already awesome, so do not detract from it with silly hair accessories.

- Choose the appropriate colour: always choose a hair accessory that resembles the colour of your hair. So, if you have black hair, go for black or dark-brown accessories. Blue or green-coloured hair accessories are out of the awesome mane equation.

- Go for cotton or cloth-made hair accessories whenever possible: this means avoid using rubber bands from the office and don't get hair bands that have metallic bits. Cotton and cloth-made hair accessories are gentle on the hair and won't damage your awesome mane, so always choose textile-based ones.

- Consider the length of your hair: most hair accessories are best used when your hair has reached at least a medium length. Stay away from wearing hair accessories when your hair is short as most hair accessories don't serve a tangible purpose for short-length awesome manes (except do-rags).

The above 4 points should be the defining factors to consider when selecting the right hair accessory. Abide by them and remember: when in doubt, don't wear hair accessories!

These are the details of the specific hair accessories that I recommend for your awesome mane:

Headbands

These are bands that are wrapped around your head to pull the hair back. They are ideal for those times when you are doing some form of physical activity and need to have a clear visual field (i.e. your hair doesn't block your eyesight). Headbands are very popular among male sportsmen such as soccer and tennis players, and headbands can be used in social settings too.

Use headbands when your hair is at least a medium length. Stick to headbands made of cotton or other textile material and choose those that are no wider than an inch. Stay away from plastic headbands and blend the colour of the headband with your natural hair colour.

Hair bands

Also known as hair ties, hair bands are the smaller version of headbands, and they are used to tie the hair into a ponytail, braid or bun. They are very useful to secure the hair when you need the most assurance that your hair won't be moving around. Hair bands also work great for when the occasion calls for a neat look with long hair (e.g. in the workplace).

Hair bands should be used when your awesome mane is at a medium or long length and can be tied. Again, choose the hair band according to the colour of your hair, and avoid hair bands that have metallic bits in them.

Bobby pins

These are discreet and thin metallic pins that are useful for securing your hair in place without making it look like you have anything in your hair. They are best used when your hair is at a long length, and you should only use a few at a time. Bobby pins take some skill to master, and I recommend you to ask any females whom you know about how to use bobby pins since most ladies use them or know how to use them. It is imperative that you choose bobby pins that match your hair colour as they should not be visible at first sight.

Do-rags

The do-rag is a fitting piece of cloth that is used to cover the scalp and is useful for preserving your curls from daily wear and tear as well as for any instances where you will be rubbing your hair against anything (including on a windy day). The bandana is similar to the do-rag, only that the former tends to be less fitting around the head than the latter.

Unlike the previous hair accessories, do-rags can be used with any hair length, including near-shaved.

Hair picks

Also known as afro picks, hair picks should be used mostly by those with an Afro hairstyle (Type V curls). This is because the great volume of the Afro hairstyle in Type V curly hair allows for the hair pick to be held in place; no other hairstyle or curl type can hold a hair pick in place like the Afro in Type V curls hence the hair pick's specific use. The hair pick is very useful to retouch one's Afro and detangle any formed knots, and it has become a fashionable item to sport on one's mane provided that the hair is such curl type and in such hairstyle.

Putting everything together

Identifying your curl type, measuring your 2 hair lengths, finding your optimal shampooing frequency, knowing what hairstyling agents to use, choosing a suitable hairstyle, knowing how to shop for a good barber; your eyes are probably dry from all the reading and digesting of information you've done so far in all these chapters. Not a problem; you have embarked on a journey to mane awesomeness, and there's no need to rush it.

The next chapter will be dealing with the mental part of achieving and sporting your awesome mane, so it is by now that the physical part for your awesome mane has been covered in all chapters up to here. There will be some more content relating to the physical part of your awesome mane in the following chapters too, but what you have read till here is the core of what you should be doing to get those curls looking awesome. Continue reading this book and, when you finish, then start implementing your awesome mane actions.

The goal now is to put some form of order in which to approach the physical aspect of your awesome mane so that you can get going and start taking actions. Before putting all your newly-acquired hair knowledge into practice, however, you must be confident and positive about starting your awesome mane journey. In the following chapter, I will cover in depth the positive attitude and mentality that you should have to achieve your awesome mane, but you must convince yourself at this stage that you now have everything in your power to get your awesome mane. So, if you weren't already positive about achieving your awesome mane, then it's as simple as doing it right now: you are about to start a journey that will yield results soon and that will improve you immensely as a modern male, and you have all the knowledge needed for it in this book. It doesn't get any easier than telling yourself that last sentence a couple of times to get immensely stoked about putting yourself to action with your curls!

The way that I have structured the preceding chapters is pretty much what the flow should be in terms of starting and continuing with your awesome mane journey. This is the flow that I recommend for best results as it has you first identifying all that there is to your curly hair while building a wealth of knowledge that will then allow you to tackle the oh-so-important physical aspects of hair grooming and hair care.

Going with the recommended flow to set the path for your awesome mane, you must first familiarise yourself with all the content in the second chapter "Curly Hair 101: Know Your Waves, Coils Or Kinks" and start by implementing the acquired knowledge in that chapter as the first step of your awesome mane journey. What is to come now below these lines is the chronological order of awesome mane steps and actions that I recommend you to implement and follow for your journey.

Chronological order of the steps to take for your awesome mane actions

Step 1: Know your curl type and your hair lengths

Chapter 2 "Curly Hair 101: Know Your Waves, Coils Or Kinks" deals with the basics that have you understanding your hair so that you can then associate and make sense of the actions taken with regards to hair grooming, hair care and hair enhancements. Thus, you must have the following 4 elements worked out as the first step of your awesome mane journey: curl type, extended hair length, extended hair length category and visible hair length.

If your current hair is damaged from having used chemicals or straighteners, then get a haircut and start growing your awesome mane from scratch.

Step 2: Get yourself the hair products

After working out all the 4 elements in Step 1, move to your hair grooming. It is time to buy yourself (if you don't have already) a shampoo, a normal conditioner, a leave-in conditioner and a hairstyling agent. Use the tables in Appendix XXIII, Appendix XXIV and Appendix XXV to work out which hairstyling agents suit your curl type and hair length. For the shampoo and conditioners, simply get conventional ones: a shampoo with a sulfate-type ingredient, and the 2 conditioners with any of the ingredients listed in Question 7 of the Q&A chapter "Questions & Answers: Because They Will Come". Don't make it overly complicated, your goal for now is to be as basic as it gets when it comes to hair grooming products.

Also, ditch any hair brushes or conventional combs that you may have. From now on, your only hair-manipulating tools will be your fingers and a wide-tooth comb. Purchase a wide-tooth comb that is either metallic or wooden, avoid plastic ones. You can buy at this stage a hair dryer if you want, but you will not be using a hair dryer until you have your hair grooming routine sorted out; you can buy the hair dryer later on in your journey as it won't be of use for quite some time.

Step 3: Know your natural hair for a week

Before finding your shampooing frequency and making use of your conditioning and hairstyling agents, you will go on a 7-day mission to know your natural hair. To start this hair-learning week, shampoo your hair the night before and then commence this special week the next morning; during the upcoming 7 days, you will not shampoo again, nor will you use anything else on your hair. Essentially, every day of this 7-day period will be a non-shampooing day, and you will only be performing the Sebum Coating method and your preferred hair-drying method, which will thus allow you to get some good practice with both these secondary actions.

Your goal in this introductory week is to pay attention to how your hair reacts so that you can see for yourself how it dries on its own (i.e. air-dries) from damp to fully dried and how your curls look naturally, all while familiarising yourself with the Damp vs. Dry effect and, overall, getting a good feel as to how your hair behaves without any added products or manipulation. Your mane will not look its best during this week, but take this period as a week-long lesson on your own hair. Once the week is over, shampoo your hair and perform the next step and set of actions.

Step 4: Find out your optimal shampooing frequency and learn to style your hair

Knowing your optimal shampooing frequency is paramount.

Concentrate on finding out your optimal shampooing frequency and take your time. Use the generic guidelines as explained in the hair grooming chapter (and as seen in Appendix XXII) during the period that you will use to find out your optimal shampooing frequency: use a normal conditioner only on your shampooing days, do the Sebum Coating method and use a leave-in conditioner on your non-shampooing days, and apply your chosen hairstyling agent every day whether it is a shampooing or non-shampooing day. Stay with only 1 hairstyling agent until you have found out your shampooing frequency.

Start practising the styling of your mane concomitantly as you find out your shampooing frequency. Familiarise yourself with your chosen hairstyling agent, get used to styling with your fingers or wide-tooth comb and grease the groove of drying your curls, whether it is with a towel or via the Shakeout method. Avoid using hair dryers for now.

Finding out your optimal shampooing frequency may take you up to 16 weeks as you will be assessing every 2 weeks the state of your mane. Take your time, don't rush it; you will be seeing vast cosmetic improvements in your mane as you get closer to your optimal shampooing frequency.

Step 5: Know your conditioners like you mean it

After having experienced the importance of your optimal shampooing frequency as you took the time and effort to find this particular frequency, you can now experiment with your normal conditioner frequency as well as with the frequency of use of your leave-in conditioner. Just like with shampooing frequency, give yourself some weeks to ramp up and find out your optimal frequency for both normal and leave-in conditioners although you can start using the leave-in conditioner every day without slowly ramping up the frequency if you so wish; leave-in conditioners offer great benefit when used daily as a hairstyling agent anyway.

For your normal conditioner, a good starting point is to use it on 50% of your non-shampooing days. For example, if you are doing 1 on/6 off for your shampooing frequency, then start by using the normal conditioner on 3 of those 6 "off" days (i.e. 50%); do remember though that you will also be using a normal conditioner on your shampooing day by default.

Use the same 5 indicators used to assess your optimal shampooing frequency to now gauge and fine-tune your response to an increased conditioning frequency (normal or leave-in). Likewise, use the same trend of reviewing your hair every 2 weeks as you advance towards your optimal normal conditioning frequency, only that you will now be inserting the secondary action of "using a normal conditioner" on an extra non-shampooing day of your hair grooming schedule. If your hair is looking too greasy, has tiny white particles breaking off or is still looking dry, then adjust the frequency of use of your normal or leave-in conditioner while leaving the shampooing frequency unaltered.

As a general rule, you will find that using a normal conditioner on your shampooing days and doing the Sebum Coating method plus using a leave-in conditioner on your non-shampooing days will, many times, suffice in terms of optimal conditioning for your awesome mane. Thus, start with such conditioning frequencies until you secure your optimal shampooing frequency, and then, if you want to play around with a higher normal conditioner frequency, use the "50% of off days" rule; if you want to play around with a higher leave-in conditioner frequency, introduce the leave-in on 50% of those days in which it isn't used or alternatively ramp up the frequency as you desire.

Step 6: Master the 9-Minute Perfect Mane routine

Only when you are acquainted with the 3 hair grooming stages and their main and secondary actions, will it be time to become efficient at synchronising the stages to define your daily routine (i.e. the 9-Minute Perfect Mane routine). Basically, your goal is to master your hair grooming routine, aiming to get to those 9 golden minutes of your daily hair grooming time. Don't rush the process of becoming efficient with your hair grooming routine; in the beginning, you will quite possibly take +20 minutes to finish your day's worth of hair grooming, don't worry about this. Merely worry about being determined to cut down the time that it takes you to finish your daily hair grooming, getting there slowly but surely, a few seconds less per day that passes.

The goal is to get your hair grooming routine down to 9 minutes, not because this is the mark that defines an awesome mane or because that will give you extra curly hair wizardry skills. Not at all. Getting your routine down to 9 minutes will mean that you have learnt to maximise the time-managing component of your hair grooming and can then fully reap the convenience factor of an awesome mane. For example, the 11 minutes that separate a 9-minute hair grooming routine from a 20-minute hair grooming routine can become crucial when you have to wake up early to go to work and you try to avoid getting stuck in rush hour traffic. And let's not forget that those 9 minutes that make up your hair grooming routine imply not only convenience but also great-looking curls.

The template for the 9-Minute Perfect Mane routine as laid out in Chapter 3 "Hair Grooming: Get Those Curls Looking Great" is the one for a typical shampooing day, which is the day that determines how the rest of your weekly schedule flows. Thus, your 9-Minute Perfect Mane routine changes secondary actions on non-shampooing days, yet the flow of stages and emphasis on the 3 main actions is at all times preserved. Always remember: you must clean, condition and style your awesome mane regardless of the day it is.

Step 7: Get your proactive and reactive measures sorted

The cool thing about your hair care is that you can start applying all your measures right from the very beginning of your awesome mane journey; you can work on some, and you can leave others for later. However, once you have your hair grooming routine mastered, it is time to fully address and maximise your hair care measures and strategy.

The 2 issues of dry hair and tangled hair will already be addressed, and just about be optimised, by your hair grooming, so any added hair care measures for these 2 issues at this point will be the icing on the cake and will integrate together with the rest of the hair care measures that you were carrying out by default via your optimal hair grooming. Because you will have already got into the habit of optimising your curly hair by having addressed its grooming first, any hair care measures that you now start implementing will too become second nature, which will possibly be in contrast to how much you dreaded these measures when you first read about them in Chapter 4 "Hair Care: Looking After Your Healthy

Awesome Mane". For example, tying your long-length curls at this point will make much more sense and be more welcomed than when you first read about this measure.

As for hair loss, you will be noticing increased shedding due to the enhanced slip from the conditioners and your natural sebum; really, the only thing you should be doing is investing in a vacuum cleaner to remove the shed hairs from the floor.

It is also a good time to be aware of your hairline and look into your family history for any signs of male patter baldness (MPB). Part of having an awesome mane is appreciating your curls and being aware of a hair loss condition that goes with being a male, as is MPB.

The advice on my nutritional approach for an awesome mane can be applied whenever, just make sure that you stick to it long term to truly benefit from ingesting the optimal nutrients for better hair and overall health. Since this nutritional approach will affect not only the looks of your hair but also your health (for the better), you must consult your doctor prior to making any changes in your diet and/or nutritional supplementation, and it would be wise to also have a general health checkup to know your current health state and be able to compare it with any future checkups. Ask your doctor; he/she will be able to tell you what you need to do and get checked. Just like your barber or hairdresser, your doctor is another ally in your quest for an awesome mane.

Your hair care measures and your nutritional approach compose your hair care strategy, or, in other words, by addressing these 2 essential elements of your hair care, you will have created the approach to looking after your hair over the long term. Your hair care strategy is dynamic and should be reviewed from time to time; your hair care measures will require some minor tweaks as your hair length changes over time.

It is once your hair grooming is in order and is being executed optimally that hair care must then be fully addressed and maximised. Ultimately, these 2 aspects of the physical part of your awesome mane (hair grooming and hair care) are what will tangibly build your awesome mane.

Step 8: Enhance that awesome mane

Once you reach this step and have performed all the previous steps and necessary actions, you will have achieved the physical part of your awesome mane. Anything that you do by now will consist of finishing touches because the grounds for your awesome will already be established.

All you have left is to give your awesome mane its form and shape. Trying and testing different hairstyles, choosing the right barber to get suitable haircuts, deciding whether to purchase hair accessories, merely going solo with the Shake & Go in terms of hairstyles; they are all options that should be considered at this point of your journey.

Be creative, test and experiment; curly hair has an important experimental component that is quite awesome because each head of curls is different: you will have a curl type, 2 hair lengths, a coil factor, a high or low density of hair strands, thick or thin hair shafts, secrete a lot or too little sebum, and, of course, there is a one and only you. The stuff that flourishes atop your head is just another piece of the puzzle that makes you, and you can most definitely use and customise this piece to your advantage; never forget that, my friend.

Reaching the awesome mane destination

You will have achieved your awesome mane when you are satisfied with your hair and with how it suits you in the grand scheme of things. The next chapter will cover the mental part of your awesome mane, and it will show you that your awesome mane will be achieved when you have fitted your curly hair into your self-puzzle and to the person you are as a modern male. This mental part is an on-going process during your journey that starts with the right attitude, but, in terms of the great looks of your hair and the physical aspect of your awesome mane, the flow that I recommend for starting and developing your awesome mane journey is pretty much as described in the previous subsection's 8 steps.

With all the practice that you will get during your journey, the daily management of your awesome mane will soon become second nature, and, when it is the time to change anything (e.g. hairstyle or shampooing frequency), you will be able to do so with no inconvenience on your part and still sporting an awesome mane. It is all your acquired knowledge and hands-on experience during this journey that will be determinant in having an awesome mane lifelong and without dramas. Look at it over the long term, and understand that the uniqueness of your curly hair implies a certain amount of experience (i.e. awesome mane journey) prior to fully knowing and mastering those curls.

My personal experience

I soon realised that I first needed to master the grooming and caring of my curly hair before I could consider enhancing and putting the final touches to my then to-be-acquired awesome mane. Metaphorically speaking, I could not see my journey as putting the cart before the horse despite most of the stuff I would read about hair would in fact sell the cart without even considering that there need to be a horse too!

My curly hair does best with a Shake & Go approach at short and medium lengths, and I have rocked my mane with a Shoulder Length when it was long, having also grown my curls to beyond chest length and approaching the navel. To enhance my experience and knowledge, I have experimented with plenty of hairstyles and lengths during this past decade, and, due to the hard-to-tame nature of my coils, I have been able to learn plenty on all that relates to styling and managing curls.

When it comes to barbers, I find that shopping around for one whom you can trust and rely on is the best option. I avoid going to hair salons that have too much decoration and that look like tea houses, and I have walked out of a barbershop on more than one occasion because the barber failed to listen to me and be professional. Upon achieving my awesome mane, I quickly learnt to appreciate my hair, which meant that I no longer settled for just about anyone cutting my hair. In fact, I once grew my curls long because I had moved to a new country and I just didn't trust any of the hairdressers in my new city.

For hair accessories, I use headbands and hair bands frequently when my hair is beyond a medium length. They are very useful when I am lifting weights (my sport is Olympic weightlifting) or being otherwise physically active. Both headbands and hair bands are very easy to lose though, so I tend to buy a big stash of them every couple of months. I don't use any other hair accessories as I like to keep things simple and prefer my awesome mane to be rocked au naturel for most of the time.

My awesome mane journey started very much like I have recommended you to start yours. As you will learn in the next chapter "The Mental Part: Attitude, Lifestyle And Making It Awesome", I had to rehash the attitude to my hair and to my life, and, being still a teenager, I saw this as the perfect opportunity to continue improving my self-puzzle and grow as a young adult. The mental part of your awesome mane is being ingrained in you as you read this book, and the next chapter will be decisive to fully solidify the right mentality required to sport great-looking curls.

Without further ado, let's continue now with the mental stuff!

The Mental Part: Attitude, Lifestyle And Making It Awesome

"Toughness is in the soul and spirit, not in muscles"

Alex Karras

In this chapter, I will go through everything related to the mental part that is inherent to being successful in your awesome mane journey because you can buy all the magic hair products that you want and make all the resolutions that you may so wish to, but, if you don't have the attitude, the inspiration, the motivation and the determination to integrate your awesome mane into your life, you will not last long with your precious head of great-looking curls.

To oppose the dead rats and the buzz cuts, a change in attitude is in due order. You have already read what the attitude to an awesome mane entails: embrace that which is inherently yours (your curly hair) and do something positive about it. I had to ingrain this same attitude in myself in order to successfully take the first few steps of my awesome mane journey because I had to literally change the perspective that I had on my hair from negative to positive. After all, my curly hair would keep on growing curly whether I liked it or not, so I had 3 options: a buzz cut, a dead rat or get my act together and fix this problem. I picked the third option, and I soon realised how I had to develop a positive attitude around my hair that would incidentally carry over to the rest of my life.

For best results, your awesome mane should be seen as part of enhancing yourself as a male. We all share the desire to be better men, and the actual process of achieving great-looking hair allows one to maximise what I term the "self-puzzle": those traits that, when put together, make you who you are as a unique individual. You are not just getting your curly hair looking awesome; you are improving as a male living in a 21st century modern society.

Indeed, it is the attitude and form of thinking that an awesome mane implies that can also be projected and carried over to other areas of your life so as to continually improve yourself and self-actualise. Once you have achieved your awesome mane, you will have got your curly hair done and dusted (i.e. turned a weakness into a strength) and will have developed the confident attitude and habits to ensure that it remains awesome for the rest of your life, so now, what do you do next? Well, you use the positive momentum created from having accomplished this follicular goal to continue improving other areas of your life.

On another mental part note, having an awesome mane also requires inspiration. We curly dudes just plainly lack the inspiration to do something about our locks. From celebrities to the average Joes you see every day, you will be lucky to count with the fingers of 1 hand those dudes whom you remember making enough of an impression on you to inspire and motivate you to really want to make something positive of your curly hair. You can go back in time as far as you want, you'd still have spare fingers left in your hand after counting your historical sources of inspiration and motivation. This sought-after awesome mane inspiration, which I will cover later on, plus the knowledge that you have acquired with this book puts you in a great position to make the most of something that is yours and that had long been neglected.

All of the above is why there's more to an awesome mane than just an optimally-groomed and properly-cared head of curls. See this occasion as a time to start a "positivity ball" rolling with regards to your life. We can all improve different areas of our lives regardless of how petty or trivial they may be (e.g. hair), and, by starting with adding one success in the form of an awesome mane, you can jump-start a momentum of positivity and keep it rolling by tackling and optimising other areas of your life that require an improvement.

As your usual in this book, in this chapter I will be emphasising ad hoc how all the content has related to me because, now more than ever in <u>The Curly Hair Book: Or How Men Can Now Rock Their Waves, Coils And Kinks</u>, you need to realise that what you are going to embark on is the right step in the right direction of a life that is aimed to be full of achievements and successes. Furthermore, I will be constantly reiterating the self-puzzle concept and how it relates to your awesome mane because my experience has taught me that it is only when one gets to see the self-actualising side of his hair, that the awesome mane journey can be finished and accomplished.

The attitude to an awesome mane

Striving for your awesome mane will require an effort from your side, and that effort will not only be limited to the grooming and caring aspects of your curly hair. You will have to defy conventional notions, have to think differently and have to actually achieve your goal; all while blending your newly-discovered appreciation for your hair into the self-puzzle that makes you who you are as an individual. That's some awesome effort that you are going to be putting into your hair, so you will need a strong attitude and mental foundation.

As you will remember from the section "The 5 Rules To An Awesome Mane" in the first chapter "Introduction: The Start Of An Awesome Mane Journey", the right attitude to have consists of positivity, determination and assertiveness, qualities that are endogenous to all successful people and that can be worked on by any male no matter his history of successes in life.

When it comes to positivity, you have to start by regarding your hair as a positive asset of yours, which is easier said than done but is absolutely doable. With this book, you have all the knowledge that you need to make your curly hair look its best, so change your attitude to your hair now. Stop reading for a moment and go now to the closest mirror you have; look at the reflection of yourself and of your hair, and say this, "this is me and this is my hair, and

I'm about to make my hair look the best I can". As cheesy as it may sound, try it; you'll be surprised at how it will make you see that, indeed, your hair is how it is and that you now have the power to improve and control the stuff that by default grows on your head. You are not trying to convince yourself that you can be an astronaut or that you can buy a huge mansion; you are trying to tell yourself that the stuff that you are looking at directly is absolutely and 100% improvable. You don't even need convincing because you already know that you can do it from having acquired all the knowledge in these previous chapters.

Whenever I have curly haired dudes coming to me for hair advice, one of the things that most of them tell me is how much they hate their hair because of how bad it looks. Well, no surprise Sherlock, if you hate something, you will never try to make it look good! Lack of knowledge and inspiration is behind this lack of trying to improve one's curly hair, and it only takes a man to know how to actually fix a problem to begin addressing it. Thus, learn about your hair, and you will be on your effortless way to improving it.

When I tell the aforementioned curly men that they should start finding their optimal shampooing frequency, that they naturally secrete a natural conditioner that should be spread along their locks (i.e. Sebum Coating method), that they should not be using hair brushes to style their curls, and the many more knowledge gems that you find in this book, these same men rapidly begin to notice how their curly manes begin to look better upon putting words into actions, and their perspective on their hair changes just as rapidly; they no longer hate their hair and, instead, embrace it. In your case, you have in this book all the knowledge needed to get your curly hair looking awesome, hence the easy part of your journey is actually embracing your hair and being positive about it. Rest assured, your hair will soon look awesome, and it will become a highly-valued asset of yours.

When it comes to determination, you must be 100% sure that you want to do this. Do not give it a half-baked or lazy effort because it will not work, and you will not obtain your awesome mane. You must be aware that your awesome mane will require some trial and error from your part such as when finding your optimal shampooing or conditioning frequency. You have the templates, the routine, the steps and the detailed information, yet you must regard this as an evolving journey that will also be pleasurable as you continue advancing and seeing the results of your efforts.

You will see results within a few weeks of putting your acquired knowledge into practice, but it will take some time for you to carve your hair into your own style, personality and self-puzzle. Once you get your hair grooming, hair care and the rest of physical tidbits sorted, you will literally open the door to a new you as you'll be able to grow your awesome mane long, wear it short or do a Shake & Go and be out of the bathroom in minutes. The cool thing is that not only will you see fast results as soon as you start you awesome mane journey but you will also have fun and you will be once and for all at peace with your hair.

Lastly, the assertiveness part of the attitude to an awesome mane implies being a man. A real man, not one of those pseudo males that the likes of those MTV programs try to embed in our minds. As you start building your awesome mane, you will be noticed by others, and this means being asscrtive in your actions. You may sometimes feel down or feel that your self-confidence is running low; take a look at yourself in the mirror when this happens and see what you have achieved with your hair: it looks great, you have done it all yourself, and you have taken something that is naturally yours and changed it from negative to positive while the rest of men go about their lives with dead rats and buzz cuts. Seeing what you have so far achieved with your hair will instantly smooth out any low moments during and after your awesome mane journey.

Ultimately, your awesome mane will be tied to your own self-puzzle, which is the personal puzzle that makes you as a male; never forget that. You have done it all yourself so keep your chin up because if you have had the guts to make the most of something that is going to be there with you for the many years ahead, and, by default, you have accepted to carry it with you everywhere you go, then you can certainly tackle anything else that is put in front of you. It is this boosted confidence in yourself, in knowing that you are making the most of your self-puzzle that is of the utmost value. Be assertive during your awesome mane journey and thereafter: I am the first one who believes in you because I have gone through the same that you will now go through, and it takes a real man to turn a weakness into a strength.

Integrate your awesome mane into your own self-puzzle

Every one of us is different in our own ways, but there is something that we all share, and that is trying to be the best we can. Your own self-puzzle is made up of your physical and mental traits; in essence, it is the combination of these traits that makes you who you are as a unique individual, and you can think of your self-puzzle as what someone who knows you very well would say to describe you. At all times, we seek to maximise this self-puzzle in one way or another, and your hair is one of those traits that adds to the portraying of who you are as an individual. The vast majority of curly men do not take advantage of this follicular trait, and, only when they address it, do they get to see the magnitude and potential of that which comes to them naturally. In my case, I'd say that the ability to enhance my self-puzzle via my awesome mane was one of the most-unexpected benefits during my journey.

An awesome mane is awesome because it is tailored to your desire and fitted according to your peculiar self-puzzle. You now have the knowledge to make the most of your hair, and you will be carrying your hair proud and with the right attitude; all you will have left to do is to customise your curls to the person you are! Perhaps you are a senior executive in a big company and prefer a classic look for your Type II curls, then the Side Swept will look great on you and will exude that self-confidence of yours. Or perhaps you are a teenager and want to really get to know your Type V curls while growing them very long, then get yourself an awesome Afro growing for the time being and maybe purchase a cool hair pick. So many options will be available to you once you get your your awesome mane going that the enjoyable aspect of achieving your awesome will be customising it according to your self-puzzle.

When integrating your awesome mane into your self-puzzle, there are 2 main issues that must be considered: dropping any stereotypes with regards to looking after your hair, and making the mistake of allowing your hair to construct who you are instead of the other way around.

First of all, being stereotyped is a big worry for many curly males, and it causes them to go about life without truly taking advantage of the stuff that populates their heads. It so happens that we have been led to believe that convenience and being a male cannot go together with curly hair; instead, we have to either succumb to a buzz cut or, for those thrillseekers, sport a dead rat. Always remember the assertiveness part of the attitude to your awesome mane; do not be put off by fears of being stereotyped because an awesome mane will obliterate any fears you may have as you will actually get to see how others will appreciate both your hair and the guts you've had to pull it all off. The proper hair grooming routine, fine-tuning your hair care strategy and knowing a few extra bits and pieces while carrying the right attitude is all you need, for you are achieving your awesome mane to fit and fill in that piece of your self-puzzle that has been missing for so long, not to be a hair-obsessed diva who drinks tea in hair salons.

Secondly, some men make the mistake of constructing their own selves through the hairstyle that they choose. Typically, this is done as part of a fad or trend, or to fit into a group. There's absolutely nothing wrong with wanting to belong to any urban tribes or social groups as there is also nothing wrong with emulating the latest hairstyle that your favourite celebrity is sporting. However, achieving an awesome mane requires you to think for yourself and not be a sheep; it allows you to customise your hair so that you can have your core self bettered. Never use your hair to define who you are: use your own self-puzzle to customise your awesome mane and use the synergy achieved to further define yourself as a male.

By integrating your awesome mane into your self-puzzle, you are gaining an advantage over the rest of average Joes. Not only will you improve your looks but you will also be gaining more self-confidence and will be able to polish your desired image as a modern male who has his own needs and wants, yet shares with the rest of men the commonality of wanting to maximise his self-puzzle. Whether you are a busy CEO who can only afford 10 minutes in the morning to groom his curly mane, a bohemian artist who relies on bouts of inspiration to create art or a regular guy merely wanting better hair, the goal of an awesome mane is to have you finally embracing your hair so as to fit this integral piece into your unique self-puzzle.

Check out the following examples of popular curly haired men:

- George Clooney (Type I curls)

- Adrian Grenier (Type II curls)

- John Turturro (Type III curls)

- Corbin Bleu (Type IV curls)

- Will Smith (Type V curls)

What do the men above have in common apart from being successful males? They all have integrated their curly hair into their self-puzzles. These guys are walking around with their awesome manes and have succeeded in life; they are perfect examples of what it means to have an awesome mane, and they certainly illustrate the end result of adequately fitting a great-looking head of waves, coils or kinks into one's life and personal core.

Do you think George Clooney would have hit it off as an actor had he been sporting a dead rat instead of the awesome mane styled in a Caesar Cut that he had during his acting career in ER? I was only a kid when Mr. Clooney was becoming famous worldwide as ER was televised globally, and I remember women drooling over the dude and his emblematic Caesar Cut while men were quick to try and copycat his hairstyle. Or how about Will Smith, didn't he sport some fresh hairstyles as part of his defined cool self-puzzle during The Fresh Prince of Bel-Air? Do you think Will Smith would have been as popular among young dudes (myself included) had he left his Type V curls cropped in a buzz cut during all seasons of The Fresh Prince of Bel-Air?

What, not enough examples of what it means to blend a great-looking head of curls into one's self-puzzle? Allow me to add a few more popular curly men with a bit more detail:

- Type I: Hugh Grant in the movie 4 Weddings and a Funeral. Solid middle-parted waves.

- Type II: Matthew Morrison, great looking Ivy League hairstyle in the TV show Glee.

- Type III: Justin Timberlake in the film The Social Network. Justin showing what a talented curly dude he is as not only can he sing but he can act too.

- Type IV: Troy Polamalu in any of his matches before he puts his helmet on. A gentleman on and off the field, Troy sports long kinks that make him stand out graciously.

- Type V: Lenny Kravitz in the video clip for his song "Believe". Lenny has sported many hairstyles for his Type V kinks during his career, serving as a great example of what can be achieved with this curl type.

Then, you also have those average Joes who have embraced their curly hair as part of making themselves overall better men. Have a look at my website, you will see examples of men from all over the world who have followed suit with their awesome manes, each one of them coming from different walks of life.

You want a guy with a PhD in Biomedical Sciences who sports his waves while he is photographed in the Great Wall of China? Or how about a busy London-based manager who keeps his coils looking neat and classy as he goes about his day dressed in a suit? And the guy with long awesome Type IV curls resembling those of Troy Polamalu and who has been to remote places such as Shibuya in Tokyo? Or how about me, a curly haired dude who has lived in 5 countries, lifted over 300 pounds over his head while sporting a six pack and has been the first man to have a website for curly men (and on top of that write a book on the topic!)?

All of the examples above, illustrating both popular and average Joes, represent how great curly hair can look, what the attitude should be to have an awesome mane and how one's curly hair should be fitted into one's self-puzzle. Nothing more, nothing less; these men have ultimately become better males because they have chosen to turn a perceived weakness into a strength. And you, my friend, are already on your way to becoming another example.

Social references for an awesome mane

If you think about it, it is not entirely our fault that we curly men lack any desire to do something about our curls and grow an awesome mane. We just don't have enough social cues and references to get inspired by and try to emulate.

The hair care industry is dominated by a straight-hair perspective, and, despite the industry being primarily driven by female consumers, this same perspective spills into the men's hair niche. Straight hair is, simply put, much easier to be managed and put into submission than its counterpart: curly hair. Women (and men, to a point) are brainwashed to straighten their waves, coils and kinks so as to copy the latest trendy celebrity sporting manageable, smooth, silky and straightened hair. Men with curly hair are told to keep it short and tamed and to focus on other attributes to build their physical appearance. But, why have to avoid something that when managed properly will improve one's core as a male?

Most men go about life spending their hard-earned money on exorbitant gym memberships, weird facial-grooming gadgets, silly abdominal-toning-sculpting machines, overpriced clothes, extravagant and sometimes toxic perfumes, and frequent visits to the barber to make sure that their curly manes are tamed and forgotten. If some of that effort was diverted into doing something positive about their hair, then we'd be talking awesome mane town, and we'd have plenty of sources to become inspired by and be motivated to act by!

153

So yes, it is difficult to find social references these days with regards to sporting an awesome mane. I know this because a good part of my hair-learning efforts have been dedicated to finding these social references. It is, in a way, sad to see that we curly men are not as privileged as our straight haired peeps in finding sources of hair reference and inspiration on a daily basis. We men have great sources of social reference and inspiration when it comes to building a body, building our wallets or choosing what career to take, yet the awesome mane part is extremely undeveloped.

If you look hard enough, however, you will be able to find famous and popular men to obtain your source of awesome mane inspiration from. Moreover, with this book, I am confident that our awesome mane ranks will increase steadily so that we get the word out, act and inspire. Remember our silent gentlemen's agreement from the 5 rules of your awesome mane? With your new curls and attitude, I am trusting you to inspire others in any way possible, something that you will be doing by merely going about your life with an awesome mane. But first, you yourself need to achieve said awesome mane, and I am 100% confident that you will achieve it and go on to serve as yet another example of what it is like to carry a great head of curls as a modern-day male.

I have already mentioned in this chapter a good amount of celebrities with awesome manes according to their curl type. Because I want to ensure that you can fully relate to the self-puzzle concept regardless of your worldwide location, allow me to now bring you even more awesome mane sources of inspiration, but this time listed per continent!

- <u>North America</u>: Steven Bauer, Denzel Washington, Eduardo Verastegui, Will Ferrell, David Hasselhoff.

- <u>South America</u>: Edgar Ramirez, Gonzalo Valenzuela, Diego Peretti, Sergio Torres, Ronaldo de Assis.

- <u>Europe</u>: Michael Fassbender, Paolo Maldini, Ruud Gullit, Cary Grant, Joaquim de Almeida.

- <u>Asia</u>: Saif Ali Khan, Shahrukh Khan, Imran Abbas, Hrithik Roshan, Nicholas Saputra.

- <u>Africa</u>: Omar Sharif, Taribo West, Majid Michel, Tumisho Masha, Andrew Abalogu.

- <u>Oceania</u>: Russell Crowe, Eric Bana, Jay Laga'aia, Tana Umaga, Digby Ioane.

- <u>Antarctica</u>: Sir Ernest Shackleton (well, he was a explorer and spent a good amount of time there!).

What's even greater is that the above men not only have awesome manes but they have also lived great lives. They are unique and unrepeatable men who have been leaders, pioneers, motivators, references and explorers, and, by default, they have transferred their attitude to life to their waves, coils and kinks. They have great curly hair, whatever their type, and they are also men who can be looked up to and be inspired by when it comes to living a successful life.

In addition to the above, the attitude required to achieve an awesome mane is the same that is required to succeed in life (i.e. positivity, determination and assertiveness), and this life-enriching attitude in itself is also lacking heavily in terms of sources of inspiration. In today's world, we have too many popular pseudo males acting as social references who don't do us men a favour when it comes to setting a good example of what a man should be like and of what a solidly-rooted and unique self-puzzle should be built as. From men who are utterly obsessed with their looks to men who have forgotten what it is like to be a gentleman, young (and not so young) men grow up and live their lives being bombarded on a daily basis with plenty of attitudes to life that one could argue are not the best for establishing the grounds of being a confident and successful male.

Forget about "bling-bling", about "hoes" and about "Playstations" for a second, and try to remember when was the last time that you saw a male on TV or a magazine whom you and your male ancestors would have agreed was a prime representation of a man. Yeah, finding only one is surprisingly difficult now that you actually think about it, isn't it? If we can't find a couple of popular gents to regard as references to look up to and be inspired by when it comes to being an authentic male, how on earth are we then going to be able to find an inspiring dude with a great head of curls paired with the right attitude? Sure, David Beckham, the insignia of the modern male (as the ads would want you to believe), has some great (straight) hair, but this same guy spends some absurd amount of time styling his eyebrows because his wife tells him to do so! I'll personally pass on him being an inspiration to me of what a real man should be like, thank you very much.

Do not be put off by the apparent lack of awesome mane examples in today's society. On the contrary, see this as extra motivation to go ahead and get your awesome mane and set yourself apart from the rest of men. Our lack of awesome manes and inspiration is fuelled by the lack of confidence that most curly men have to address their hair and to be themselves. Acquire your awesome mane to further enhance your self-puzzle, be yourself and set the example for others. There's more to life than dead rats and buzz cuts!

How to achieve your awesome mane

It's beautifully simple: you will have achieved your awesome mane when you are satisfied with your hair. Earlier in this book, I mentioned that an awesome mane doesn't understand of age, race, lifestyle or whatever you may think is a valid excuse to not make the most of your curly hair; being satisfied with your hair is the primary goal of an awesome mane and each one of us can do it. The day you look at yourself in the mirror and say, "I am happy with my hair", will be the day when you will have achieved your awesome mane. This satisfaction in your hair will not only come from how it looks but also from how it has been exquisitely fitted into your self-puzzle: the physical and mental aspects of your curly hair are at stake in achieving such specific satisfaction.

The order in which to start your awesome mane journey is not that important. You can pretty much start with any of the specific bits of knowledge that you have learnt in all these chapters. A good start and flow for your journey, though, would be as recommended in the previous chapter: do all the profiling and identifying of your curly hair first (i.e. curl type, 2 hair lengths and length category), then move to mastering its grooming through your routine, followed by applying the hair care measures and building a strategy, and finishing your journey by making the final enhancements of what is now your awesome mane.

What is really important is that you start acting on the physical part of your awesome mane soon, don't delay it. The mental part of your awesome mane is being built as you read these lines: you are both consciously and subconsciously encouraging the positivity towards your curly hair as you read this book, and the optimal attitude is being ingrained in you as you are acquiring all the knowledge needed to succeed in the journey that you are about to embark on. You will only be able to sustain the drive to start your awesome mane journey for so long before the drive vanishes and you end up losing interest; hence, the need for you to act soon and ensure the early start of your awesome mane journey.

It is once you start your awesome mane journey that a constant stream of positive results must then be sought by implementing specific steps and actions as outlined in the last chapter. The goal is to maintain the long-term motivation needed to continue your journey since being motivated will be crucial to achieving your overall goal of an awesome mane. In other words, not losing your motivation during your awesome mane journey should be your main priority. Allow me to elaborate on this in the paragraphs below.

A goal, whatever it may be, is achieved by implementing over the long term a series of goal-oriented actions that yield a constant stream of positive results. When it comes to actually achieving the goal, one must maintain his motivation throughout the entire journey as motivation is what fuels the desire to continue working towards achieving the set goal. Motivation throughout the journey to achieve the set goal is reinforced by the constant stream of positive results from the goal-oriented actions that one implements.

The specific goal-oriented actions that are implemented during the journey yield said constant stream of positive results. These actions and their consequent positive results can be regarded as the smaller pieces of a puzzle, with these pieces ultimately making the puzzle that would be the set goal. As one progresses in his journey to the set goal, seeing the hard work (i.e. goal-oriented actions) paying off (i.e. positive results) is what will have one waking up every day motivated to implement one more action to get closer to his goal.

The initial wave of motivation and energy that has one desiring to start the journey to the set goal is created from inspiration. By becoming aware of the specific benefits that someone else enjoys from having achieved a goal (i.e. inspiration), one will then desire those same benefits for himself too and will become stimulated to achieve the goal that will bring about those benefits (i.e. motivation). Basically, inspiration coming from social references acts as the catalyst for the whole process of achieving a set goal.

This concept of goal achievement can be applied to any other goal in life, not just an awesome mane. Visually, it looks like this:

<u>Figure 25 – How to achieve a goal</u>

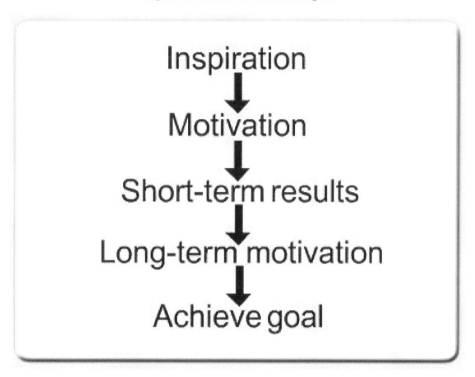

The above concept is why I emphasise so much being inspired and having social references when aiming to fulfil and achieve the goal of an awesome mane. Inspiration creates the initial motivation to achieve the set goal, and it is this newly-created motivation that gives one the drive to act. However, humans are not patient by nature, which means that one must be rewarded in some way sooner than the time that it would take to achieve the set goal. Thus, one must be rewarded with a constant stream of positive results obtained from implementing specific goal-oriented actions; all of this fuelling and reinforcing one's long-term motivation. And motivation plus the right knowledge and tools is what will have you achieving your set goal.

I realise that I'm starting to read like a psychology textbook and that it seems quite obvious that I have a thing for puzzles, but stay with me throughout as the mental part of your awesome mane is just as important as the physical part. Let's now apply the above goal-achieving concept to your awesome mane.

157

You may not be motivated to do anything positive with your curly hair because, in a nutshell, you haven't been inspired yet. You haven't seen anyone whose mane would be worth emulating and who motivates you to pursue an awesome mane so as to reap the same benefits that he has obtained from having addressed his curly hair optimally. You have yet to find a fellow curly haired male with an awesome mane who not only has great hair but also has women drooling over him, a great career, a great body or has helped make the world a better place. Instead, you may regard those with great-looking curls as diva-like and self-centred, and I would not blame you if you did indeed think like this before you started reading this book.

Read this whole chapter again from the very beginning and start identifying your sources of inspiration. If the names and examples of men that I have used still don't serve to inspire and motivate you to achieve an awesome mane, then stop reading right now and leave your house in this very moment. Keep your eyes wide open because your goal is now to find at least one male who not only has a good head of curls but who is also an inspiration to you for whatever reason.

As weird at it may look, approach a fellow curly man and start chatting with him in a friendly manner. You may find, for example, that he is a married man who works 2 jobs to ensure that his children have their basic needs covered. That itself is worthy of admiration and inspiration. You may find another curly haired dude who is a bachelor and is in great shape and health, and every weekend he hooks up with the hottest women; that could also be of inspiration to some! See the objective? Look beyond the physical part of hair, and see for yourself that an awesome mane is the result of a particular attitude to enhancing one's self-puzzle; an attitude that separates the winners from the losers and one that breeds superior men.

You being inspired is enough to spark the motivation to achieve an awesome mane, but, to really keep the spark going, you must also have an intrinsic desire to do it. This intrinsic desire is shared among men in that we all want to maximise our self-puzzles; we all want to be better. Your newly-found inspiration plus your innate desire to be better can then ignite the motivation to turn a desire into a specific action: to start your awesome mane journey. By all means, you may currently be at a stage in your life in which immediately starting your awesome mane journey may not be ideal, but, sooner rather than later, this intrinsic desire will kick in naturally, and all it will take will be for you to be minimally inspired to get fired up to achieve your awesome mane. When this happens, though, do not delay the starting of your journey as your fired-up drive will only last a limited amount of time.

By now, you have plenty of awesome mane knowledge to start putting into actions, and you will find that each goal-oriented action will add yet another positive result to your journey. The gradual accumulation of positive results will then maintain your long-term motivation, allowing you to cruise through your journey and ultimately achieve your awesome mane.

Finally, the attitude than an awesome mane requires will serve to ensure that, when the going gets tough, you stick to the plan and pull through. Your attitude is ingrained in you because you already know for sure that you can achieve an awesome mane no matter what: you have the knowledge and the inspiration, and you can now regard your curly hair as a problem that can be fixed. Once you achieve the goal of an awesome mane, you will be required at times to tweak its maintenance (e.g. a change in shampooing frequency due to a change in lifestyle), but your already acquired knowledge and experience will enable you to react smoothly to any changes that need to be made, always rocking your awesome mane regardless of any tweaks or changes!

An awesome mane is sexy

The sexiness of an awesome mane is enough to warrant a section dedicated to how much its sexy side is appreciated. After all, since we are dealing with a physical trait that is instantly recognised by humans, I might as well give you a very good reason to strive for its achievement. Women (and men) find an awesome mane to be uber sexy and achieving a great-looking head of curls will enhance your attractiveness greatly. This is a fact and is quite welcomed, though it should not be your primary reason to achieve your awesome mane. Allow me to relate below to how an awesome mane will enhance your perceived attractiveness by using my case as I have experienced.

I have chatted with plenty of women in many countries during my international travels, and I have carried out my fair amount of, let's call it, "field testing". Regardless of culture, country or language, each and every woman that I have met has expressed the same attraction to curly hair. Upon meeting me, all women without exception would express their appreciation for my awesome mane: from asking me how I look after it to mentioning how "luscious" my curls look because they are well groomed. This has not been intentional for I haven't purposely achieved my awesome mane to have women drooling over my curls; instead, the fact that all these women have appreciated my curls has been a mere side effect of striving to better myself as a male and improving something that is part of my self-puzzle.

It is not that women solely love curly hair or that I am the curly version of Brad Pitt. Not at all; women also love straight hair or even a shaved head, and I am certainly not the most good-looking guy in any given bar or room. It is not the texture of the hair specifically that makes women love curly hair; rather, it is the confidence that an awesome mane exudes that gets their panties wet.

Women are used to seeing curly haired men with dead rats on top of their heads or with very short and tamed inexpressive manes. Women are not used to seeing a luxuriant head of curls, and any man who takes the step to be different and acknowledge what he has as a male will win plenty of extra points when it comes to attracting the opposite sex. You will literally stand out.

You see, women love confidence. They love how a man evaluates a situation and takes the right actions. They love how a man grabs his life by the horns and succeeds. They love how a man expresses his uniqueness, carries himself proud and sets himself apart. Does this sound familiar? With your awesome mane, you will be walking around with yet another proud asset of yours, showcasing the world your confidence in yourself. Not only do you have the great-looking hair but you also have the attitude and self-confidence, a steamy combo that works great to attract women.

There is even a biological reason for the above. Many of our physical traits as humans are designed to advertise to the opposite sex our ability to survive and reproduce. In men, physical traits such as wide shoulders, powerful backs and buttocks or an ability to grow strong and healthy-looking hair act as cues to subconsciously attract women. Way back in the days when men didn't have Playstations to waste their lives with and humans had to rely on their physique and instincts to survive, assets such as hair or physique shape allowed men and women to rapidly gauge the ability of a potential mate to survive and reproduce. Even to this day, this subconscious attraction to specific physical and personality traits is still very palpable. Women desire men with athletic physiques, thick-looking hair and self-confidence to top it all (to name a few desired traits). On the other hand, we men want women with healthy-looking long hair, wide hips and firm breasts. It is not that both men and women are being irrationally picky; no, the reason for this is that our brains still rely on cues such as hair to assess a good candidate to reproduce with (play doctor and nurse in the bedroom) and pair with (get married and have children) to pass on our genes.

The reality is, women love confident men, and you will gain heaps of self-confidence if you stop being like the rest of male sheep and instead study, learn and apply all there is to an awesome mane. Likewise, the vast majority of us don't have all the qualities that make the absolute perfect man (in fact, there's no perfect man as there is no perfect woman), yet all of us curly dudes grow atop our heads a trait that can be totally revamped and added to our list of qualities; a list of qualities that every woman will be subconsciously going through when deciding whether to get jiggy with you or not.

Start taking care of your curls and get your awesome mane integrated into your own self-puzzle, then see how you reap the sexual benefit of having made the most of what you have as a modern-day curly haired male. Guaranteed!

The benefits of an awesome mane

After having just given you above a pretty good reason to achieve your awesome mane, it is more important, however, to put your awesome mane into context with your everyday life. What will be the specific benefits that you will obtain after having achieved your awesome mane?

Self-confidence

As I have said a good number of times already, your confidence in yourself will skyrocket. Not only will you improve your looks and feel better about yourself, but the fact that you have achieved your awesome mane and the fact that you have turned a weakness into a strength will prove to yourself as well as remind you that you can achieve anything you set yourself.

Personal satisfaction

Achieving goals leads to a sense of well-being, and the achievement of your awesome mane will be no less. You will feel good on a deep, personal level; no longer will you look in the mirror and see your hair as the stuff that needs to be cropped and forgotten about. You will have taken a step to improve your self-puzzle, and that is in itself a powerful source of personal satisfaction.

This personal satisfaction and the boost in your self-confidence that will result from achieving your awesome mane will allow you to carry both your hair and yourself with pride. The great Aristotle best described pride as "the crown of all virtues", meaning in your case that pride will result from achieving your goal of an awesome mane and from possessing an attribute that is worthy of admiration as it was obtained via those same traits (i.e. virtues) that are essential to success in life.

Be careful not to confuse pride with arrogance or use pride to put down others or lose touch with reality. You will become an overall better man by having an awesome mane, and you will need a humble element in your character to carry your awesome mane successfully for the rest of your life. The personal satisfaction that you will receive upon achieving your awesome mane is just too great on a deep, personal level to be ruining it with arrogance; you have my word.

You will learn about yourself

I like to see the achievement of an awesome mane as a micro and macro lesson in oneself. "Micro" because you will learn all about your hair, how it reacts, what to expect, how to manage it and how to make it look its best. "Macro" because an awesome mane will have you honing your qualities as a male and will be tangible proof that you can do that which you put your mind to. It only takes improving something as trivial as hair to remind you that you are a male capable of achieving great things while learning more about yourself.

You will reinforce a positive attitude

It's all about reinforcement, about wiring the brain to identify problems and seek solutions. You will reinforce yourself that a positive attitude is the first step in achieving a goal, and you will ingrain a winning mentality in yourself, which will be indispensable when achieving further goals you set yourself down the line. As I have explained when it comes to achieving goals, you will be reinforcing and ingraining in your brain the process that yields success. We humans are creatures of habit, and, the more we practise and grease the groove, the more efficient we become in our actions.

You will be regarded by others as a better version of your old self

Hair makes a good chunk of that first impression that we all make. When you walk into any scenario, people instantly notice your posture, your physique shape, your facial expression and, of course, your hair. Whether it is a business meeting or a date with someone, these 4 elements will be subconsciously analysed in a split second by others and will influence people's response and behaviour to you. It is a bizarre aspect of life, and the reason why the "first impression is the one that counts".

For those who already know you, an awesome mane will be regarded as an indication of the trust that you have in yourself and will positively change the perspective that your acquaintances had on you. I know guys who have been promoted at work upon fixing their curls and making use of the same attitude that is the basis of an awesome mane. It is actually quite fascinating how we can influence others by the way we look; talk about still having a primitive brain!

You will inspire others

It is human nature to look up to others when it comes to achieving goals. You were once inspired, and you will be in the near future a source of inspiration. Not just for having great-looking curly hair but also for having had the attitude, the guts, the determination and all those character traits that having an awesome mane has required and meant. Whether it is inspiring your children or inspiring some random curly haired dude who saw you walking in town, you will be a source of inspiration and motivation to others.

Inspiring others will bring you much positivity, ranging from being complimented in person by others to the personal satisfaction that you'll have of knowing that you are walking around minding your own business while helping other curly men realise that having great-looking curly hair as a male is doable and possible. The vast majority of fellow curly men only need a spark, a source of inspiration, a "seeing for themselves that it can be done" to acquire that drive and motivation to improve their curls, so you will be inspiring others without even saying a word. The first time that you are complimented in person will be awkward in a good way and will further boost your self-confidence; be prepared to have not only women but also men complimenting your head of curls!

Lastly, while you will have your ego stroked quite a few times from having a visible head of great-looking curls, try to always strive to inspire and help others. It will be very easy to turn your self-confidence and pride into arrogance, so try to stay with your feet firm on the ground and remind yourself of the difficulties that those who you have inspired may have. Not every male has the same knowledge or ability as you have to achieve an awesome mane, and it is a good reality check to be aware that you are privileged to even be physically able to strive for an awesome mane. Life has an amazing way of rewarding those who help others, and you will obtain plenty from being a source of inspiration to others.

An awesome mane is part of an awesome life

Yes, this book is about achieving great-looking curly hair and grasping the right attitude to manage it as a 21st century male. However, I cannot ignore, as I write these lines, the fact that we are also modern males in societies that are hectic, competitive and stressful to live in. Aiming to become better and better is not an option, it is a must; and, when aiming to improve our self-puzzles via our hair, we must also think holistically. In other words, there will be synergies created when you achieve your awesome mane, and I would like for you to at least be aware that you will be able to build further improvements and achievements in your life upon achieving your awesome mane.

Let me reiterate that an awesome mane is not about turning you into a hair-obsessed diva, and it certainly isn't about emphasising and prioritising your hair above all else. If you did this, you'd be a fool; a sad fool, for that matter. I can assure you that when you embark on your awesome mane journey and start seeing results, you will get a sense of well-being and personal satisfaction that will be worth every minute of your hair grooming and hair care. This is because you will be tangibly feeling the enhancement of your self-puzzle via the improvement of your curly hair, which will then increase your self-confidence, improve your looks and ultimately better you as a male. However, don't just leave it at that; don't just be a man who has great hair and also, well, just great hair.

We can all improve different areas and aspects of our lives, from apparently-trivial matters such as hair to important issues such as relationships or one's career. Once your hair has been improved and you have achieved the goal of an awesome mane, you will start a positivity momentum going on. This means that you will be enthusiastic and open to continue improving yourself since success breeds further success: just like you were enthusiastic to improve your hair because you had developed a positive attitude around it, you will now be optimistic and feeling positive to further improve yourself because you will have already accomplished a goal and you can see the results of it in the mirror. Take advantage of this situation.

I speak from personal experience and from the experience I have helping others; you will find the positive environment and self-confidence created from achieving your awesome mane to be of great use to continue tackling other aspects of your life that need improvement. You will have sparked the motivation to continuously seek life improvements and the enhancing of your self-puzzle. Heck, there is even research showing that testosterone levels increase dramatically after achieving a goal and being triumphant; you will literally have more of that hormone that makes you a man once you achieve your awesome mane!

The premise to this life-bettering concept is to start first with the smallest and easier-to-improve areas of your life to get the ball rolling and encourage positivity, for achieving your set goals and improving the smaller areas in your life will build and encourage a success-seeking and positive mentality. Thus, once you achieve your awesome mane, you can move on to other areas that are a bit more important in your life such as, let's say, your physique. Then, once you achieve this further goal (e.g. better physique), you move on to improving even more important areas of your life such as communication skills, relationships or career, and so on and so forth. Start small, think big, and keep the positivity rolling.

Using the explained concept above, this is the positivity flow you'd encourage with the examples used:

Figure 26 – Visualisation of the process for long-term positivity

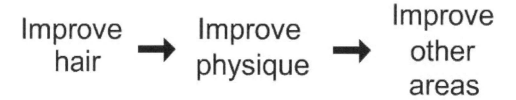

By all means, the next area in your life to tackle as part of improving yourself as a male can be anything other than physique, I just happen to have personally used this transition to help others, and it goes smoothly. You can work on whatever you deem necessary after your awesome mane; it doesn't matter, what matters is that you are now in a position to continue milking the positive momentum created from initially addressing your dead rat/buzz cut. Next you know it, accomplishing goals will have become intuitive and a habit.

Of course, hair and physique are just 2 pieces that make your unique self-puzzle and that make you who you are; there's plenty more that you can tackle as a next goal to achieve once you get into this life-bettering habit. And while I am aware that it is easier said than done, ideally we should all be emphasising the enhancement of our self-puzzles with concomitantly living life to enjoy it.

From looks to personality to career to family, this explained life-bettering concept is based on one continuously addressing each subpar area of his life, identifying where improvements can be made and concentrating on achieving the set goal before moving on to the next. As I say, the potential for self-actualisation (i.e. improve yourself as a whole) with the achievement of your awesome mane is too great to not be mentioned; I can only go so far to use this book to help you address your curly hair optimally, instil in you the right attitude to have for your hair and provide you with the same concepts and ideas that have helped me in my life so as to not only have an awesome mane but also a better life. You and I share the same desire to become better men and enhance our self-puzzles, and an awesome mane will be your one step forward towards a better life. That's a given.

You live your life however you wish, and your priorities and goals in life are all unique to you. Having said that, the beauty of an awesome mane (no pun intended) is that its achievement creates the right environment for you to continue working on bettering the rest of your life. Because you now have the knowledge to do something about a trait of yours that wasn't a strength to begin with, you are consequently able to create the positivity and motivation needed to support your goal of improving said trait. Knowledge and inspiration are behind the lack of accomplishments that each one of us may have, and, in your case, now that you have the knowledge and inspiration needed to achieve your awesome mane, you will be able to piggyback on the self-actualising momentum that you will have created once you achieve your awesome mane.

To top it all, whatever you decide to improve next will be tackled, by default, with you already sporting a great head of curls and a derriere-kicking attitude to boot!

My personal experience

It wasn't until I had actually started the journey to my awesome mane that I realised how my goal would only be achievable if I resolved to fully change my attitude (instead of a half-baked change). My awesome mane experiments required me to be pretty much alone in my endeavours, and this required the unveiling of a certain character trait in me that was yet to be exploited to its maximum potential. Up until then, I was happy to conform to what the rest of the mass conformed to. As a guy still in his teens, my teenage friends were doing their hair as the latest straight haired celebrities were doing. My curly haired friends would buy hair straighteners and straightening products and beat their curls into submission so as to imitate the cool hairstyles of then-popular straight haired males like Johnny Depp, Kurt Cobain, Nick Carter and David Beckham (gee, I feel so old writing this). That, or these same friends of mine were "buzz cutting" their way in and out of the barbershop every 2 weeks.

Personally, the same attitude required for an awesome mane has also brought many benefits to my life. Having started my awesome mane journey at such a young age, I was able to learn how knowledge on its own won't cut it to succeed in life; a solid attitude is needed to be able to sport one's curls successfully for the long term, and this solid attitude consisting of positivity, determination and assertiveness is one that fuels a successful life.

Life is all about enjoying it too. When I was 18, I packed my bags and decided to see the world with the goal of experiencing the next coming years as an adventure. The only thing I knew for sure was that my scalp would continue to produce unmanageable (at the time) curly hair that would tangle, become dry and look like a desert bush while being an annoyance for the most part. As soon as I started experiencing this life adventure, however, my eyes were opened, and, among many enriching experiences, I got to truly learn about my hair as I experimented with it and became my hair's best expert through trial and error, consistency and determination (and some stubbornness too!).

Overall, I have tried to bring wholeness to my existence by addressing the different areas in my life through my chosen lifestyle. I have experienced, I have travelled, I have discovered, I have failed, and I have succeeded; all as part of enriching my life and making myself a better man. Thus, I can only recommend you, above all, to strive to become a better man with an awesome mane, it really is worth the pursuit.

7) Hair Mythology: Don't Be Fooled Any More

"Bullsh*t!"

Arnold Schwarzenegger

There are many myths and wrong beliefs surrounding hair. In men, curly hair has the most baloney associated to it; this being primarily engined by a lack of hair knowledge on our side (curly men) and by the hair care industry having a predominant straight-hair focus.

Part of achieving the knowledge needed for your awesome mane is being aware of the myths that accompany hair and knowing fact from fiction. Unfortunately, many hair myths continue to be propagated in this day and age despite the advent of the internet, and there is a lot of misinformation going around with hair, especially misinformation that is then used to snowball the nonsensical mythology and folklore associated with hair. Likewise, hair-related myths are sometimes spread unintentionally by average folks while, other times, myths are spread and maintained alive by those who have vested interests in them.

In this chapter, I will cover those common and not-so-common myths that surround hair and that many of us have fallen prey to at one time or another. You now have the knowledge needed to achieve your awesome mane, but it is a fact that you will encounter some hair myths along the journey, and these myths may be tempting to fall for despite your already-extensive knowledge of your hair. So, without further ado, let's kick those myths were the sun don't shine!

Myth 1 – Trimming hair makes it grow faster or healthier

I have heard this one even from hairdressers themselves, but it makes sense that this myth continues to be propagated as the more visits you make to the hairdresser, well, the more cash he makes. If your hairdresser tries to convince you to believe this myth, run for the hills.

The truth is that there is no way for a hair follicle to tell when the shaft has been trimmed. There is some evidence pointing to hair growing a little bit faster in summer, which is coincidentally when you are likely to get your hair trimmed more often as you will be outdoors and wanting to look good. Correlation does not imply causation, however, so cut your hair whenever you think it is optimal to do so and without factoring in this myth.

Myth 2 – Shaving hair makes it grow thicker

Just like with the previous myth, the hair shaft doesn't have any nerve endings to sense when it has been shaved. Your hair follicles keep producing the same amount of hair at the same rate and with the same structure whether you shave the hair or not.

Hair that has been shaved will feel thicker when it is at a very short length (i.e. near-shaved) because the shorter a hair strand is, the less pliable it will be. Furthermore, when hair is shaved, the newly-created tip of the hair shaft is formed at an angle, which further exacerbates the perceived thickening-effect and, in effect, makes each hair strand a follicular blade knife.

Take two straws. Cut one of them so that it is only 1 inch in length while the other one remains at whatever length it is (e.g. 5 inches). Now, hold the uncut straw with one hand and use the palm of your other hand to smoothly apply pressure along the length of the straw; it will bend. Now, try to do the same on the 1-inch straw; it won't bend and will feel as though it is harder. Now, image dozens of 1-inch straws placed vertically and next to each other on a board measuring 4 inches by 4 inches. That's exactly what happens with hair as it grows after being shaved: it will go from less pliable to more pliable as the hair strands increase in length. Nothing else.

Myth 3 – Hair grows from the tip

I have been surprised at the amount of people that I've found who think that this is true. The inclusion of this myth in this chapter is, more than anything else, to illustrate how profoundly unaware average Joes are about their hair. In the case of this myth, this is not entirely our fault as we are constantly bombarded on TV with hair products that focus solely on the ends of the hair strands, thus the association with something going on in this segment of our hair.

The good thing is that you already know that your hair grows from the follicle and that you are continuously producing new hair material, which actually provides a cushion for your hair caring efforts because, if you end up damaging your hair, you know that new hair segments will sprout regardless. However, don't take this as green light to go and look after your hair carelessly because hair grows 0.5 inches of length per month, and any damage to the segment of the hair strands close to the scalp can take many months to be outgrown.

Myth 4 – Plucking 1 grey hair will have 2 growing back

Not at all. If you are lucky, the same grey hair will grow back again as if nothing happened, and, if you are unlucky, you will have damaged the hair follicle from pulling the hair strand out of the follicle socket, which will lead to defective hair growth or even no more hair growing out (grey or not grey).

My advice is to simply cut the specific grey hair strand very short with a pair of scissors if you only have a few grey hairs. If you are greying around most of your head though, then I suggest that you get on with the program: grey hair can look great and can indeed enhance an awesome mane. On the other hand, you can dye your hair to conceal the greying but try to go with discreet and elegant tones that match your natural hair colour; don't make it too in your face.

Myth 5 – There is good hair and there is bad hair

This myth was in part launched into the mainstream by Chris Rock's movie <u>Good Hair</u> although the good hair/bad hair concept has been unfairly ingrained in people with Type IV/V curly hair for many decades, and, in some countries, it carries racial connotations.

The good hair/bad hair concept views Type IV and V curly hair in its natural state as "bad hair" while "good hair" is viewed as hair that is either straight or of a looser, more defined curl type.

Of course, this whole good hair/bad hair thing is a lot of baloney because any man, regardless of curl type, can get his awesome mane and thus have good hair.

In fact, if I were to dig into semantics, I would put it like this:

- "Good hair" is the equivalent of an awesome mane.

- "Bad hair" is the equivalent of a dead rat.

There are no hair textures, curl types, skin tones, ethnicities or races involved when it comes to bad hair. If you don't take care of your hair, it will be "bad hair". Plain and simple.

Myth 6 – You must shampoo your hair daily for optimal hygiene

As you know by now, the whole "shampooing daily" concept took off in the '60s with the advent of the hippie movement. As it goes, back in those days shampooing daily was cunningly associated by the big hair care companies with not being a hippy, which helped to establish the daily use of shampoo when decades earlier, shampoo was used with lower frequencies and with less-processed ingredients.

As I have covered so enthusiastically in this book, reducing shampooing frequency is the best way to go for an awesome mane. From skipping shampoo every other day to shampooing once a week or even once every couple of weeks, you will have to play around a little to find your best shampooing frequency. Make sure that you fully understand how to find your optimal shampooing frequency and that you know what to do on the days that you do not shampoo because your optimal shampooing frequency is key in achieving your awesome mane.

Myth 7 – You can straighten your curly hair by brushing it

Not only is this myth wrong, but, if you try it, you will end up damaging your hair. I have talked to a good number of men who, for some reason, believed that furiously brushing their curls like mad men would straighten their waves, coils or kinks. Then, when they saw that their hair turned into huge balls of frizz from the brushing, they would blame their lack of results on not brushing hard enough, thus starting a vicious hair-brushing cycle that ultimately damaged their hair beyond repair. Yes, this is the extent to which many curly men are brainwashed to reject their naturally-forming curls!

Brushing your hair will break its curl pattern and will only lead to merely pulling your hair and even pulling hair strands out of their follicles if you brush hard enough. Avoid at all costs.

Myth 8 – Straightening one's hair doesn't damage it

Because many of us have been led to believe that straight hair is good hair and that straightening our hair is just "how it is", curly men (and women) don't question the actual process of submitting their curls and changing their texture. You can straighten your hair with straightening gadgets or by using chemicals on your hair, and both methods work to physically alter the hair strands, creating damage to the structure of the hair shafts so as to be able to change its curled pattern and yield the straightened look. The hair shaft cannot repair itself, so it is better to prevent any damage in the first place than trying to repair it.

Avoid straightening your awesome mane, but, if you insist on straightening your curls, only do it very rarely.

Myth 9 – Curly hair doesn't grow as long as straight hair

This myth is partly true. Your genetic makeup is the ultimate factor that determines the final length that your hair can achieve, and people with straight hair do not have specific genes that dictate that their hair can grow longer than curly hair. However, and as I explained in the second chapter "Curly Hair 101: Know Your Waves, Coils Or Kinks", curly hair takes the longer distance by default when it grows, and one's coil factor will determine how long the hair can visibly grow to (i.e. the visible length it achieves).

All factors equal (including genetic makeup), curly hair will not achieve the same final visible length that straight hair will achieve because, despite the fact that both textures will have grown to the same extended length, curly hair will have curved and bent along the way. Having said that, you should not be worrying much about this peculiarity unless you are planning to grow your hair to navel length and beyond.

Myth 10 – Curly hair can be cut just like straight hair

As outlined in the fifth chapter "Achieving The Physical Part: Putting Your Mane Together", you should be striving to find a barber or hairdresser who has experience cutting curly hair. For the most part, curly hair must be cut in a dry state and not in a wet/damp state, which is the opposite of what a typical barber would do with straight hair (wet the hair before cutting it).

Our hair texture shrinks when it dries from a wet state, and each one of us will have his unique and specific coil factor, which makes it almost impossible to predict how the haircut will finally look when the hair dries. Most barbers and hairdressers will not think twice before wetting your hair and proceeding to cut your curls, which is the same approach that is used with straight hair.

While curly hair may be slightly dampened, especially when the majority of the cutting job has been done, you should be getting your awesome mane cut by someone who has experience cutting curly hair and who doesn't view cutting curly hair the same as cutting straight hair. You have been warned; I have experienced and seen some horrible haircut cases that stemmed from having wetted the curly hair prior to cutting it. Never underestimate the ability of your curly hair to coil back into place!

Myth 11 – Growing your hair long makes you less predisposed to balding

I have heard this one a lot. Fact is, by having longer hair, you have more hair mass on your head, which can conceal your balding, and this is where the myth comes from. If you are balding (MPB), you should treat your hair follicles with the utmost care, so growing your mane long (6+ inches) is not the best idea as long hair has a tendency to be pulled and catch on things. Last thing you need is losing more follicular soldiers in battle through unintentional pulling. Wear your balding hair at a short or medium length, elegantly and, most of all, with pride and confidence. You can have a balding awesome mane too, it's all about how you fit it into your self-puzzle!

Myth 12 – You can train your hair to be a certain shape or type

Your hair grows from your follicles as genetically determined, hence you have your given curl type. While hair texture can change at critical stages of one's life (e.g. puberty), your hair will not otherwise change how it grows just because you think you are training it. Last time I checked, for something to be trained, it needs to be able to assimilate information, process it and learn from it. You can train your dog to fetch your slippers, but you certainly cannot train your hair to grow wavy instead of kinky. Of course, you can make the most of your hair and turn it into an awesome mane, but that implies solely making your hair looks the best it can within your identified curl type.

Critical stages of one's life in which hair can change its curl type or texture include puberty, entering seniorhood, extreme distress (e.g. loss of a loved one), going through cancer treatment and taking some very specific medications that are used for serious illnesses.

Myth 13 – Men who care after their hair are girly or effeminate

I have heard this one especially from those men sporting dead rats for hair. These same men believe that taking care of your hair means spending half of your morning in the bathroom putting all kinds of potions on your hair while baking a cake in the oven as you make time to watch repeat episodes of Sex in the City. Yeah, right.

I heard this myth a lot prior to my inspiring moment back in 2001. It wasn't until after my inspiring moment that I got to learn of the idiocy of such claim spouted by those with dead rats. Sure, in the beginning, it took some time and experimenting to get my hair in order, but that's because I didn't have any sources to learn my curly hair stuff from. Nowadays, I just coast along spending mere minutes on my awesome mane every morning, and so can you now; neither your testosterone nor manhood is sacrificed in order to get a great-looking head of curls.

Oh, and women love men with awesome manes and despise dead rats. Next time you hear a dead rat owner say crap like this, smile at him as you grab your beautiful lady by the derriere and kiss her in the cheek. Hey, perhaps he'll get inspired!

Myth 14 – Curly hair cannot be managed properly no matter what and is an overall annoyance to have

Yes, I have left this one till the end. Booting this myth is pretty much the essence of this book. I remember going to hairdressers and being told to either spend my money on a silly hairstyle that would last 1 day or to go for a buzz cut or a short neat trim; same goes for barbers in barbershops. In fact, had it not been, some 11 years ago, for the barbershop episode that you read at the beginning of this book, I probably would not have been instigated to subconsciously look for inspiration while casually browsing TV a few days later. I basically turned negativity into positivity as I decided to enrol in one of the most exciting adventures of my life: the journey to an awesome mane.

Curly hair can indeed be an annoyance and be difficult to live with; the same way that driving a car can also be annoying and difficult if you have to drive a tin-looking car that is falling apart and don't know how to drive it. Yet, upgrade to a Ferrari Enzo and learn how to drive it, and the driving experience then becomes pleasurable and is something that you can incorporate nicely into your lifestyle so as to have a more convenient and enjoyable life. The same concept applies to curly hair, and the awesome thing is that you now know how to make the existence of your mane a pleasurable one and are consequently able to reap its benefits.

My personal experience

I didn't debunk these hair myths overnight. I went into the pursuit of my awesome mane knowing that there was a serious lack of information and that whatever was available was either inapplicable to my case as a modern male or just plain wrong. Through experimentation, researching like a crazy and asking questions and more questions, I gradually learnt what was good information, what was bad information and also how to differentiate the 2. I can tell you that I was the first one who used to shampoo daily when I started my awesome mane journey, but I quickly learnt that doing this was precisely one of the reasons why my curls were always frizzy and dry. So much for the "use daily" instructions in commercial shampoos.

I also at times experienced paralysis by analysis in that reading too much caused me to become even more confused and end up wasting my time. Many times, I was better off just going with my gut feeling and making decisions before my mind became entrapped in all my "ifs" and "why nots". After all, it was my hair that I was playing and experimenting with, so I could always shave it all off if I did something wrong.

The myths that I have debunked in this chapter have been the most notorious myths that I have come across and that you too will come across. These debunked myths, together with the rest of the specific knowledge you have learnt in this book, are more than enough to disregard all the silly nonsense that you may come across as you start your journey and continue with your awesome mane efforts. Furthermore, the next chapter will be dealing with questions that may arise during your awesome mane journey, so there really is no excuse by now to be falling for hair shenanigans!

8) Questions & Answers: Because They Will Come

"A wise man can learn more from a foolish question than a fool can learn from a wise answer"

Bruce Lee

If you have got to this chapter, you will have already acquired all the knowledge necessary to take your curls from a dreaded dead rat or forced buzz cut to an awesome mane. By now, you know which curly hair type and hair lengths you have, what a conditioner is, what hair grooming entails, how to go about your hair care, and you will already be stoked to master the 9-Minute Perfect Mane routine. You will be exuding heaps of positivity about your curls, and you will be on your way to joining our ranks of awesome mane dudes. I can assure you that you are about to boost your potential as a 21st century male once you start putting everything into practice and you get ready to achieve your awesome mane.

Of course, as the journey starts, questions will arise. Most of these questions can be solved by referring back to the previous chapters, yet there are some other minor questions that may arise as your awesome mane journey continues and that require to be specifically addressed somewhere in this book. Since I have been in your very same place, I know that there will be times when questions will indeed arise. Let's tackle them.

1) Why should I strive for my awesome mane?

What, you are asking this at this stage?

Ok, joking aside. You will ask yourself this question a couple of times in the beginning, and you may have already asked yourself this very same as you continued reading this book. Your answer to this question should be "because I want to do it".

You want to strive for an awesome mane because, as a man, you want to make the most of what you have; you now have the right knowledge, the right attitude and the right inspiration to fix a trait of yours that has so much potential. Before, you could excuse your way out of doing something about your curls, but now there's no escaping this. And there is no escaping this because, now that you have seen the light, you can set and follow the right path.

You are now able to strive towards your awesome mane with ease and do something positive about a unique trait of yours that is part of who you are as a whole. You can buzz your awesome mane, you can grow it long, you can style it in a myriad of ways, and you can shampoo it once or twice a week; it doesn't matter. What matters is that now you know how to make the most of something that is written in your DNA and that is inherent to you. All this without the inconvenience and associated nonsense that you once thought was synonym of sporting great curly hair as a male.

2) How long will it take me to achieve my awesome mane?

Subjectively, as soon as you finish reading this book. Objectively, it can take you up to 4 months.

An awesome mane symbolises an attitude and a lifestyle approach, and you can decide to pursue these 2 as you read this book. On the other hand, depending on how much of a dead rat or a buzz cut you have, doing everything as outlined in this book will have you noticing visible and tangible awesome mane results in as little as a week, but I rather give you a conservative time period of up to 17 weeks (4 months plus the hair-learning week) since I don't know the specific circumstances surrounding your curls, nor can I know your mindset. From my experience with others though, up to 17 weeks is all it takes unless the finding of your optimal shampooing frequency is delayed severely.

Because an awesome mane requires you to master the advice in this book so as to have your hair doing as you want it to and not vice versa, your awesome mane will require an initial period of learning and adapting that will consist of a few weeks. However, do not rush your adaptation, and see this for the long term; it took me years to nail down my awesome mane to a T, so I have weeded out all the unnecessary stuff that I went through, and a couple of weeks will pass by fast anyway. What matters is that as soon as you have finished reading this book, you will be en route to your awesome mane!

3) What if I cannot get down to 9 minutes with my hair grooming routine?

Nothing. Absolutely nothing will happen.

The 9 minutes of the ideal hair grooming routine is a mark of time maximisation and efficiency; 9 minutes as a timespan for one's hair grooming is perfectly doable by any able-bodied male, and it's in your interest to work towards gradually lowering your hair grooming time until you are under 9 minutes.

If you find that you cannot get down to 9 minutes for whatever reason, you will still be the owner of an awesome mane, and you will still have great curly hair (provided that you do the rest as outlined in this book). You will have certainly excelled at synchronising your hair grooming routine if you can get it all done under 9 minutes, but there's more to an awesome mane than taking this or that long to groom your hair every day. Moreover, your hair grooming may take longer than 9 minutes on some days despite the fact that you are good at it and can normally get it all done in less than 9 minutes. We all, from time to time, like to enjoy showering for more than 9 minutes with warm water and singing rock hits from the '80s!

In conclusion, just keep in mind that the 9 minutes for your hair grooming time is a mere objective cue that will tell you that you have become sufficiently efficient in your hair grooming and that you can then fully milk the whole convenience factor of an awesome mane. That's all.

4) What if I don't shower in the morning, how should I do my hair grooming routine?

If you don't shower in the morning, then you can do the day's worth of your hair grooming routine later in the day when you shower (e.g. after the gym); if you are showering before going to bed, then there is no point in styling your hair although there is certainly a point in cleaning and conditioning your hair. Since it is in the morning when you will typically style your hair, what you'll then do is wet your hair in the morning to style it and do your cleaning and conditioning later in the day when you have more time (e.g. during the pre-bed shower).

The hair grooming process should ideally be implemented sequentially and without a break; that is, the stages should follow each other smoothly as per the 9-Minute Perfect Mane routine. However, if you find yourself not being able to get the 3 stages implemented in one go, then it is fine to break them up so that you carry out each stage at different times of the day. Likewise, the hair grooming process is best done in the shower as it is more convenient although you can implement it elsewhere too (e.g. using water from the sink basin).

5) What if I miss a day of my hair grooming routine?

Ideally, you should be striving to complete the hair grooming process every day. However, we cannot ensure that we clean, condition and style our manes every single day for the rest of our lives. A day here and there without grooming your hair won't have any effects, but, if you start skipping days, you will certainly start to see a decrease in the good looks of your curls. Same goes for your hair care strategy: regularly skipping its daily doing will negatively affect the health of your curls.

The cool thing about our hair grooming routine is that, if you are going to be showering within the day, you can implement the grooming of your curls easily and without any inconvenience. Moreover, your hair grooming is easy to pair up with the rest of your body grooming and you'll be able to do it all in minutes. Your hair grooming will soon become second nature, and you will get to associate a quick shower with getting your curls groomed optimally.

6) Which should I do first, my hair grooming or my body grooming?

It is up to you. However, the 9-Minute Perfect Mane routine, as outlined for your shampooing day, takes into account that you do your body grooming in the 2 minutes that are used to leave the conditioner on your hair, and 2 minutes is more than enough to get your body groomed (i.e. cleaned).

Preferably, do your body grooming before your hair grooming on your non-shampooing days and also on your shampooing days if your body grooming happens to take more than 2 minutes. This body grooming preference is only so as to not interrupt the flow between the conditioning and styling stages of your hair grooming.

Lastly, any facial shaving should be done after your styling stage, not before.

7) What ingredients should I look for in a shampoo and the 2 conditioners?

Your shampoo should have at least 1 sulfate-type ingredient. These are some common names that sulfate-type ingredients can go by:

- Sodium laureth sulfate.

- Sodium lauryl sulfate.

- Sodium lauryl ether sulfate.

- Sodium dodecyl sulfate.

- Sodium monolauryl sulfate.

There are also shampoos that are sulfate free, but my advice is to first start with a sulfate-based shampoo, finding out your optimal shampooing frequency and building your hair grooming routine with such a shampoo. Then, once you have achieved your awesome mane, you can try a sulfate-free shampoo and see how it goes. Sulfate-free shampoos are weaker than sulfate-based shampoos in their hair-cleaning action, hence it is better that you start your awesome mane journey using the latter as sulfate-based shampoos tend to be more common and are more convenient to use when initially finding out your optimal shampooing frequency.

For your clarifying shampoo, just go by the product name including the word "clarifying" in the label; most of these shampoos contain a sulfate-type ingredient plus other specific hair-cleaning ingredients.

With regards to your normal and leave-in conditioners, you should be identifying in their ingredient list at least 1 of the following commonly-added ingredients:

- Glycerol.

- Propylene glycol.

- Glyceryl stearate.

- Cetearyl alcohol.

- Cetyl alcohol.

- Stearyl alcohol.

- Glycerine.

There are many functional ingredients that both normal and leave-in conditioners can have, but the ingredients listed above are the common ones used to make hair-conditioning products. Thus, when purchasing your 2 types of conditioners, aim to buy those that have at least 1 of the ingredients from the list above.

8) Why is my curl type III/IV when it is short, yet looks Type II when it is long?

Your hair follicles keep producing the same curl type regardless of your hair length, and there are no nerve endings in the shaft to allow the follicle to sense when the hair is long enough to change its curl type.

This noticeable curl-smoothing effect that you and the rest of us curly dudes experience when our hair is long is due to the weighting down of the hair once the curls reach a long-enough length, and this effect is most noticeable on Types II, III and IV long curls. Because of the inherent weight of long hair, the hair closest to the scalp will be pulled down continuously, leaving the curls in this segment of the strands in a permanent semi-extended state. Thus, the curls formed in the segment of the hair strands closest to the scalp will look smoother and looser in curl shape than the curls formed closer to the tip. On the other hand, the ends (i.e. tips) of your hair don't have any extra length to weight them down, so they will resemble what your true curl type is.

Note that this effect is most relevant when your hair starts to hang down naturally without hairstyling agents applied, which tends to be at the visible lengths of 4 to 6 inches for Type I and II curls, and 8+ inches for Type III and above. This effect is the reason for measuring your curly hair's vertical length from the tip if your hair is long.

9) Why does my hair look awkward when I try to grow it long?

Curly hair is known for growing in an awkward manner, especially when the hair is grown carelessly (i.e. the opposite of an awesome mane). You quite likely have tried in the past to grow your curls to a long length but found that your hair would look worse the longer it grew. This "awkward" phase tends to last until the curls get to hang down naturally, thus a curly male growing his mane long can stay with awkward-looking hair for 1-3 years at a time, and most males can't make it that long and prefer to chop their hair before having to endure the drama of growing beastly hair.

If you want to grow your curls long, the best thing that you can do is to start from a hair length that is fairly even all around your head. The length difference between the longest and the shortest hair segments on your scalp should be a maximum of 2 inches. For example, if your hair has been trimmed with the sides and back of your head shorter than the top and you want to grow your hair long (over 6 inches), then you'd want the hair on the top of your head to not be longer than 2 inches from the hair on the sides and back of your head.

The awkwardness of curly hair when growing it long is primarily due to our texture's inherent puffing-out nature, and having uneven hair lengths will magnify the puffing out and thus create said awkwardness. Having an awesome mane will make growing your curls long a piece of cake, but it won't fully protect you from having to endure some hair awkwardness before your curls get to fully hang down.

10) I am trying to do the Sebum Coating method, but I am uncertain about grabbing locks of hair, can you explain what I should be doing?

Most curl types tend to have discernible locks: a number (ranging from a dozen to a few dozens) of hair strands will be growing in the same direction, effectively forming locks, and thus being easy to spot the locks on the scalp. If you run your hands through your hair, you will be able to tell apart these locks as the hair strands group together and form visible "chunks" of hair. Basically, you could say that your mane is made up of many hair locks growing from your scalp, for each hair lock is made up of individual hair strands grouped together.

Sometimes, the locks are not so easy to tell, this being most common in Type I and Type V curl types. If you find that you cannot tell your locks apart, worry not, for having "visible" locks is more of an interesting occurrence than anything else; it doesn't mean that your hair needs to be managed differently. In the case that your hair strands don't seem to clump into locks, simply grab as much hair as you can in 1-inch-wide sets and run your fingers through the sets as described for the Sebum Coating method. Effectively, someone who has visible locks will be grabbing 3-10 locks at a time in each 1-inch-wide set, yet you'll be grabbing just as much hair in each set, only that you won't be grabbing what would otherwise be locks (since your hair strands don't clump into locks). In any case, this is a mere semantic issue; whether your hair strands group into visible locks or not, simply grab as much hair as you can in 1-inch-wide sets to implement the Sebum Coating method.

11) Is working on my awesome mane going to negatively affect my masculinity?

No, no and no! This is a question that I have been asked a good number of times by men who mentioned that all the curly dudes that they had seen in real life tamed their manes.

While I understand your concern about having your masculinity sacrificed in the name of great-looking curly hair, the reality is that the vast majority of fellow curly men that we see around with buzz cuts haven't done anything about their manes because they all lack inspiration and knowledge. About inspiration: look around harder, men with awesome manes are there; check my site for guys like you and I who too have awesome manes, and search around online for the men that I have referenced in the previous chapters. About knowledge, well, that's what this book gives you.

These same aforementioned men with their insignia buzz cuts have experienced the dead rat effect previously; they have had bad experiences with their curls and, overall, don't know how to properly go about their curly hair, so they automatically have a negative feeling towards it and prefer to forget about their hair by hitting the barber for a close crop every 2 weeks. This is quite a natural response: if you regard something as bad or negative, you are not going to do something about it unless you are shown the proper and optimal way to do it or fix it.

With this book, you get all your awesome mane knowledge and you get to insert this knowledge into your daily life in a convenient manner. I am the first one who avoids colourful hair salons with teacups everywhere, Mickey Mouse stuff and wasting my time and hard-earned money on hair minutiae: I go about my life with my curly hair addressed optimally and conveniently, no muss no fuss. Thus, I now pass on to you all my knowledge so that you too can do the same and can start regarding your awesome mane as an enhancement to your life. For all intents and purposes, your masculinity will actually be enhanced with your awesome mane, not impaired.

12) Can you go into more detail with guard lengths?

Guard lengths are the lengths of hair to which hair is cropped at with a hair clipper. A hair clipper is a tool that you will have seen your barber use to crop your hair very short and for which there are adjustable guards that allow the choosing of a specific length to crop the hair at. You can buy a hair clipper for yourself to use since this device is helpful in maintaining certain hairstyles that require frequent trims.

There are several manufacturers of hair clippers in the market, and some may use slightly different numbers for their guard lengths, but, on average, they stick to the following guard lengths:

- **#1:** 0.125 inches (3 millimetres).

- **#2:** 0.250 inches (6 millimetres).

- **#3:** 0.375 inches (9 millimetres).

- **#4:** 0.5 inches (13 millimetres).

Guard lengths under a #1 are also available, and different manufacturers approach their numbering differently. Don't overcomplicate it though as the length differences between guard lengths under a #1 are in 0.05 inches intervals, so, if you decide to purchase a hair clipper, just choose one that goes from a #0 up to a #4 and has the option of cropping shorter than a #0.

13) Why does it look like I shed more now that I use conditioners?

On average, males shed about 100 hair strands per day. This is a natural and normal process of the scalp, and it is part of the life cycle of each hair strand. A hair strand goes through a growth cycle that can last up to 8 years (it is genetically determined), and, once this growth cycle is completed, the hair strand detaches itself from the follicle (i.e. sheds) and typically falls off in the same moment. However, with curly hair, sometimes the shed hair strands will become trapped in the curves and bends that make up the rest of one's unshed hair strands. This is very common with curly hair, and a curly male walks around with shed hair trapped in his mane that will eventually fall off or be removed intentionally or unintentionally with a comb or fingers.

Both normal and leave-in conditioners add extra slip to your hair, which is why these products are great for avoiding hair tangles. Due to the extra slip provided by conditioners, you will find that the shed hairs, which in the past would get trapped in the curves of your curls, will now be falling off and be removed easily, both when you style your mane and when you are just going about your day. You will very likely notice more hairs than usual being removed during your grooming as soon as you start using conditioners and optimising your hair grooming routine, and this can be mistaken for unnatural hair loss. Unless your hairline is receding or you notice a marked decrease in hair density on your scalp, you have absolutely nothing to worry about.

14) Why does it look like I shed more when my hair is long?

Just like mistaking shed hairs for unnatural hair loss or balding when you start using conditioners, you may also fall for misinterpreting the natural shedding process when you grow your curls to a length that you have never had them before.

The reason for thinking that you are shedding more when your hair is longer is because you have more hair, plain and simple! I remember freaking out when I first grew my curls to a very long length (15 inches) and realised that the longer my hair grew, the more I seemed to be shedding, which of course was of worry as it could mean that I was starting to bald. The thing is, despite many years have passed since I first freaked out, I still have the same bushy awesome mane that I used to rock back in those days (touch wood, though!). Really, you will notice more shed hairs because there is more hair material to be physically seen.

15) When will my curls hang down?

The hanging down of one's curls is a milestone that many curly guys look forward to. Your curls can be made to hang down artificially before they will hang down naturally by using a leave-in conditioner as your hairstyling foundation and then adding a styling cream on top. Basically, you want to add extra weight to the hair strands to encourage the weighting down of your curls, and this is best done by using these 2 aforementioned hairstyling agents together.

However, for your curls to hang down naturally (i.e. in a dried state and with no hair products applied), these are the approximate visible hair lengths (not extended lengths!) that you will need:

- **Type I:** 4 inches.

- **Type II:** 6 inches.

- **Type III:** 8 inches.

- **Type IV:** 10 inches.

- **Type V:** +15 inches.

Again, the above hair lengths are visible lengths, not extended lengths. Take into account that Type V curls may virtually never get to fully hang down especially the hair on the top of the head. If you have Type V curly hair and want your mane to fully hang down, then it is best that you braid or lock your hair.

I would recommend you to not obsess about your curly hair hanging down. The above timespans are conservative (as with all growth estimations for curly hair), and, for the most part, your hair will have to be at a long length to fully hang down. Instead of obsessing about this minute aspect of your awesome mane, focus on embracing your curl type's ability to puff out, and aim to make the most of your curly hair, no matter what its type or length may be.

16) Man, why do my curls puff out so much?

This is not only a good question but also a very common question. First of all, the curving and bending nature of our curls naturally predisposes our hair to puff out; that's the way it is, and the sooner you accept this, the better. Your curly hair will continue to puff out until it reaches a length that it can hang down as per the previous question. Essentially, there is a period of length, which commonly falls under the medium-length category and is what I called the "awkward phase", where the hair will puff out the longer it grows until it hits the specific length in which it will hang down. Some funky hair drama, huh?

The good news is that an awesome mane will puff out, correct, but it will puff out awesomely. Your curls will be tamed and the puffing out will be controlled via your hair grooming and hair care. Don't view puffy hair as bad; we've been brainwashed to buzz our curls and straighten our beasts, and you and I know very well that that's not what an awesome mane is about. If your hair continues to puff out when you achieve your awesome mane, then so be it: you are taking good care of your hair and you are managing it daily, and that's what matters.

Like I say, an awesome mane will have you controlling your puffiness, but you must bear in mind that curly hair is innately puffy albeit with different ranges according to one's particular hair strands. Thus, achieve your awesome mane and walk proud with those luxuriant curls, even if they puff out!

17) Why is my curl type different now from when I was a boy?

Many curly haired men find that their current adult curl type is different from the curl type they had as boys. This is believed to be due to the effect that the puberty-induced increase in levels of sex hormones has on the development of hair follicles although the precise mechanism of action for this is not known. After puberty, a big percentage of curly haired males move up in curl type instead of moving down (e.g. from Type I to Type II).

184

My beast was a beautiful, soft and bouncy Type II when I was child. Then, I hit puberty, and my hair turned into a bushy beast of Type III and IV curls; I also transformed heavily all over my body, so the transformation of my hair was one of my lesser worries (I had a beard at age 12 that all the older guys in my school were jealous of).

18) Can I shampoo daily?

Yes, you can, especially if you have near-shaved hair. Even if you have longer hair, you can shampoo daily, but my advice to you is to then use a sulfate-free shampoo or weaker hair-cleaning products if you want to shampoo daily. Bear in mind that you will have to adapt your hair grooming schedule to this preference in shampooing frequency.

19) What if my hair gets very dirty due to a specific occasion?

If your hair gets very dirty from a specific occasion such as going camping or being in a closed room where people smoke, you can schedule a shampooing session and treat the session as if it were a shampooing day (i.e. follow the shampooing with normal conditioner and style with your hairstyling agent). Resume your normal shampooing frequency the next day; that is, the shampooing of the previous day will reset your weekly schedule.

If, on the other hand, you get your hair dirty on an occasional basis or in a frequent manner, then adapt your shampooing frequency to such. A typical scenario is playing contact sports such as wrestling, you'd certainly want to shampoo your hair after a wrestling session or any other contact-sport session. On the other hand, you don't need to shampoo if all you have done is gone to the gym and haven't rubbed your head against benches or mats. So long as your hair isn't rubbing against anything dirty, you don't have to schedule specific shampooing sessions.

If you go to the swimming pool, then I advise you to treat that day as a shampooing day; thus, deem such an activity as a hair-dirtying one since chlorine from the swimming pool is left as residue on your hair. A trick that has worked for me and for those who have tried it under my advice is to, before jumping in the swimming pool, first completely wet your hair with tap water (e.g. from the shower next to the swimming pool) and then rapidly coat your hair in conditioner (with either a normal or leave-in conditioner); you'll then be ready to hit the pool. I find a leave-in conditioner is more convenient for this trick as you can buy some leave-in conditioners in spray form or small-package form. After the swimming pool, try to do the hair grooming process (as a shampooing day) before your hair dries completely from the pool's water. This same trick applies to seawater too (e.g. going to the beach), although you can skip the wetting of hair with tap water and the soaking with conditioner since seawater is much less harsher than swimming-pool water (simply do a shampooing session when you get back from the beach).

As an alternative method to using shampoo for the above, you may use baking soda and vinegar to clean your hair on those specific occasions that your hair has got dirty. The method itself to using baking soda and vinegar as cleaning agents is detailed in Questions 32, but, in a nutshell, you can clean your hair with baking soda and then with vinegar (instead of with shampoo) for such specific hair-dirtying days, and you don't need to follow the baking soda/vinegar with a normal conditioner (just move on to your styling stage when the vinegar is rinsed).

20) Do I have to use nutritional supplements for my awesome mane?

Not at all. Nutritional supplements are only recommended so as to bulletproof your diet and have an optimal nutritional approach. Because nutrition is so important to sustain an optimal and healthy growing of hair strands, supplements allow you to provide nutrients to your hair that you aren't otherwise providing in sufficient quantities via your diet. One of the disadvantages of being a modern male is that many times we don't eat the healthiest and most nutrient-dense foods, thus nutritional supplements are very useful so as to make sure that we are not running low on any nutrients needed by the body and the follicles.

Overall, the most important part of your nutritional approach is your diet, not your supplementation, and you can certainly skip the use of nutritional supplements.

21) Isn't whey protein a steroid or dangerous?

No. Whey protein has been given a bad reputation because it is used by bodybuilders to up their daily protein intake. Bodybuilders already have a bad reputation, as it is, for taking steroids (another myth; not all take steroids), thus anything that they ingest is deemed by the general public as dangerous.

Fact is, whey protein on its own is an awesome supplement since it is basically powdered milk protein without most of the lactose and fat. Hence, whey protein is an extremely useful source of high-quality protein (a scoop can deliver 10-20 grams), and it is tolerated by those with lactose intolerance and those following a weight-loss diet. Whey protein doesn't contain steroids, illegal stuff or harming substances, and it is a safe supplement that is used by many sedentary people to increase their daily protein intake in a convenient manner.

A scoop in the morning with your milk is an awesome way to start the day, and most whey protein supplements taste delicious. Like I have advised so enthusiastically throughout this book, do consult your doctor prior to taking a whey protein supplement or making any changes in your nutritional approach.

22) What should I do if my hair is at a near-shaved length?

At near-shaved lengths, you can get away with not being as disciplined with your hair grooming and hair care. I'd still advise you to follow the methods and approaches of this book, for the hair that is currently at that near-shaved length is your current awesome mane and will be part of your future awesome mane were you to grow your hair longer. Moreover, it is best that you get used to having an awesome mane as soon as possible.

23) I am the mother/father of a boy with curly hair, should I do anything differently?

First of all, allow me to show you my admiration for having purchased this book with the intent of seeking a follicular solution for your child. It is critical to show one's son at a young age that his hair is part of his self and of who he is. As a boy nears puberty, he starts to realise that his hair is different to the hair of his peeps, and he may start regarding his hair in a negative manner as at that age boys don't like to be different. Furthermore, most parents prefer to buzz their child's curly hair because they (parents) don't know how to manage their son's curls, which further aggravates the negativity and even hate that a young boy may develop towards his curly hair.

You are the pillar of your son's self-embracing. His hair is part of who he is, and the sooner he learns to manage it with your help, the sooner he will understand his curly mane. Remember, humans fear that which they don't understand, so imagine permanently fearing a dead rat at such a young age.

The only difference with regards to his awesome mane is that you will be providing his hair management for the time being, and I recommend you to slowly get him to do his hair grooming and caring by himself. On top of that, I recommend you to not overload your son with hair products: use a baby shampoo, a mild conditioner and a mild leave-in conditioner. For his styling, use the leave-in conditioner itself or small amounts of a hairstyling agent. Of course, it goes without saying that hair products should only be used at an age in which he is aware of himself and of his hair; if your boy is in his early childhood, only use a baby shampoo to clean his hair and anything else that your paediatric doctor may recommend.

Lastly, since curly hair is genetic, be aware that you run a high probability of having more curly haired children if you or your partner have curly hair (even if only Type I aka wavy hair). Furthermore, if you have daughters, you can essentially use the same content in this book to manage their curls, though you can certainly take your girls from time to time to a tea house (aka flashy and fabulous hair salon)!

24) Can I use this book if I have straight hair or recommend this book to someone with straight hair?

Absolutely. Just about everything in this book is also applicable to straight hair; I wanted to write a book that not only had a physical part but also a mental part, and the latter is a much-needed part for curly men. Because I have curly hair and because I have gone through everything a male with curly hair has endured and will endure, I have written this book for you and the rest of curly men with waves, coils and kinks as I want you to know that having a great head of curls as a modern male is possible.

Someone with straight hair reading this book should think of his hair as being Type I curly hair, that's really all.

25) What should I expect from the opposite sex with my awesome mane?

Questions, a lot of questions. Women will flock to you for hair advice; that was the first thing I noticed upon getting my awesome mane. I have had ladies randomly popping out of nowhere in supermarkets, nightclubs and cinemas to ask me a hair question. Initially, the extra female attention is good for stroking your ego and for practising the ancient art of seduction, but it soon grows old as it becomes a daily thing. Of course, always strive to help others regardless of the gender and aim to be part of spreading the awesome mane word.

In terms of the enhanced attractiveness from achieving an awesome mane, ever since I started my site and started spreading the word online, I have continued to get the emails of men all over the world contacting me to thank me. They thank me because they see how their game with the opposite sex (or same sex) improves substantially: women are more open to flirt with them, the bedroom conversion (i.e. going from flirting to the bedroom) is pretty high, and, when they walk into a room or bar, women turn their heads to them.

I have written this before in this book, and I will write it again: women love confidence. Whether you have waves or kinks for your curly hair, a bald head or a bushy long mane, women love the self-confidence that a man emanates from having embraced what he has and from having stuck to his principles and beliefs. By getting yourself your awesome mane, you are telling people, right there and then, that this is what you have and that you are damn proud of it. This, my friend, is what gets women wet in that special place.

Work on your awesome mane, and then proceed to work on other aspects of your life. Integrate your awesome mane into a life full of achievements, and your self-confidence and male status will skyrocket; I guarantee you that.

26) I am balding/have started to bald, what do I do?

Two things: embrace it and do something about it.

Embrace your baldness. This means that you should accept that the hair will eventually go. Don't be one of those guys with a combover or with 3 hairs hanging from a ponytail. Deluding yourself will not make you look good in anyone's eyes, not even in your own eyes. Embrace your balding and be positive about yourself; at the end of the day, it is hair, and balding doesn't affect your health, nor does it mean that something is wrong with you. Balding is part of being a male, and about 65% of men are balding profusely by age 60. It will happen to the majority of us sooner or later.

Once you have accepted and embraced your balding, it is then time to do something about it. First of all, start with the hairstyle: no combovers, no long hair, and certainly no hairstyles designed to extravagantly conceal your balding.

If you are a Norwood 3 or less (i.e. you don't have big balding areas), you can still pretty much sport any of the short and medium-length hairstyles available to non-balding folks although I would encourage you to go for hairstyles that retain length at the front so as to elegantly conceal the receding occurring at the temples. Pay close attention to the term "elegantly"; this means that, when styling your awesome mane, you should allow the hair to smoothly and discreetly hover the receding temples; do not make it look like you are trying too hard. Great hairstyles to elegantly conceal the receding hairline include the Side Fringe hairstyle, the Faux Hawk, the Afro/Jewfro and the Caesar Cut. All of these hairstyles share the same short to medium-length trait and the emphasis of the hair at the hairline hovering over the receding temples in a discreet and elegant manner.

If you are a Norwood 4 or above, go for a short-length trim or buzz, or shave it altogether. At this stage, you will have too much hair-shaft thinning and balding going on at the top, which will only work against your image were you to have your hair longer than a short length. If you don't want to shave your hair because it requires doing it frequently, invest in a hair clipper and go for a #1 up to a #3 all around your head. Cropping your hair like this can be done rapidly and by yourself in the comfort of your own home, so it will be very convenient for you.

Aside from the hair, work on your self-confidence. Lose the emphasis on the hair and instead emphasise other physical attributes of yours. Look neat and polished at all times (including your remaining hair), improve the health of your skin, keep your nails trimmed and clean, brush your teeth frequently, and, last but not least, improve your body. This last one is of special importance because it will not only improve your attractiveness but will also improve your self-confidence and help you to forget about your balding.

Working on your body and getting yourself an awesome body when you are balding is what I call "pulling a Vin Diesel". While Vin Diesel himself is not the best actor around, the man exudes self-confidence and has totally revamped the public's attitude towards balding men for the better. Vin Diesel is a confessed gym addict and looks great, which coupled with his stage persona and self-confidence has garnered him an absurd amount of female followers. Seriously, Vin Diesel appears time and time again on the "hottest males" lists that all those women's magazines love to entertain their readers with, and he shares this privilege with the likes of George Clooney, Matthew McConaughey, Adrian Grenier, Will Smith and Justin Timberlake. Other men who have "pulled a Vin Diesel" include Jason Statham, Dwayne Johnson (aka The Rock) and Bruce Willis, so, really, get your awesome body and don't worry about your balding!

Lastly, I have covered the options available to fight against male pattern baldness in the chapter "Hair Care: Looking After Your Healthy Awesome Mane", so make sure that you have read these options and understood them. Do remember that currently (as of 2013) there are no options available that will yield permanent and irreversible anti-balding results outside of a hair transplant, and the latter doesn't guarantee said permanent results either. Minoxidil and finasteride only fight MPB for as long as the medications are used; if you stop using them, you will go back to balding, and you will lose any hair that had grown back.

27) I can't seem to identify my curl type, what should I do?

As I have already said in the second chapter, the vast majority of the content in this book is applicable to all curl types. However, and as you have seen so far, there are some tidbits that require differentiating the curl types, thus you should be doing all possible to identify your curl type as explained to you in Chapter 2 "Curly Hair 101: Know Your Waves, Coils Or Kinks".

If you seem to not be able to identify your curl type, then use the examples of curly men referenced in each of the curl types; all you will have to do is to search online for images of these men and then try to match your curl type to any of them, using the already found-out information that you would have retrieved from your curl typing efforts. Typically, when you find that you can't identify your curl type, you will be unsure between 2 of the 5 types, hence helping yourself with images of the referenced men will aid in identifying your curl type.

If you find that you cannot measure the vertical length of your curls, then I suggest that you try again and really emphasise the 2-dimensional view of your hair, taking photographs of your curls if need be. If you still seem to not be able to measure the vertical length of your curls, then ask a friend or family member to do the measuring for you since, many times, all we need is a fresh pair of eyes to break any visual plateaus. If you still find that measuring said vertical length is not possible, then use the examples of men referenced in each curl type while remembering that Type I and II curls form as waves, Type III and IV curls form as coils and Type V curls forms as kinks (i.e. very tight coils or Z-shaped curls).

Lastly, if you cannot measure the vertical length of your curls because you simply lack the equipment (i.e. a ruler and a mirror from which to have your head a few inches away), then delay your curl typing efforts until you have access to the equipment, and, in the meantime, you can continue implementing other actions for your awesome mane journey.

28) Can I use Arabic numerals instead of Roman numerals for the curl types?

No. Use Roman numbers (I, II, III, IV, V) as per the Curly Hair Type Guide. This is because using Arabic numerals (1, 2, 3, 4, 5) will lead to confusion as you will not be able to relate to our curl typing guide were you to interact with others or search around for related information on it.

The Curly Hair Type Guide is innovative in its nature, and I created it to provide a starting point to defining a curly male's hair grooming; hence, the use of Roman numbers was done to instantly recognise the meaning of each curl type. By now, you have learnt enough about your hair, so there's no need to be creating confusion, much less from something as straightforward as is the nomenclature of the Curly Hair Typing Guide.

29) Why is there no mention of hair relaxing and hair straightening in this book?

Because this book is about making the most of your genetically-determined curly hair. Relaxing and straightening your hair will ultimately damage it, and your awesome mane efforts will go down the drain over the long term.

With straightening your hair, you will simply be putting a temporary patch to your real problem (i.e. lack of hair knowledge) while getting hooked on the stuff as your damaged hair will only be responsive to more straightening and will look awful when you don't straighten it. On top of that, straightening or relaxing your curls is time consuming and inconvenient, for you have to know what the weather will be like for the day if you are venturing outside of your house.

This book tackles the problem from the very root: you will make the most of your hair because you have now learnt how to manage it and because you have now built an immense positivity and attitude around it. Instead of sporting a dead rat on top of your head and thus resort to straightening your curly hair, you are now able to sport a proud awesome mane; a great-looking head of curls that is all yours and that is the result of embracing yourself.

Nail down your 9-Minute Perfect Mane routine, dominate the Sebum Coating method and optimise your hair care measures; all of these put together will give you a better and more sustainable option than straightening or relaxing your curls will ever give you.

From my experience, men who straighten or relax their hair do so because they haven't learnt how to take care of their hair optimally. If you feel like straightening your hair for whatever reason, then absolutely feel free to do so, but at least do it because you now have other options to consider too.

30) Is it possible to not use any hair products on my hair?

Yes, it is. I have gone through periods of using no hair products and found this to work for my awesome mane. This solo approach is done with the same cleaning, conditioning and styling stages, only that you'd skip the actual shampoo, conditioner and hairstyling agent, solely working the Sebum Coating method for your hair grooming actions.

If you want to go hair-product solo, you would clean your hair with the mechanical action of your fingers during the Sebum Coating method, you'd condition your hair with your secreted sebum and you would style your mane in your chosen hairstyle without using a hairstyling agent. For what is worth, optimally-spread sebum works as a surprisingly-good hairstyling agent too.

This solo approach to hair grooming works best on short-length hair although you can try this approach at any length. Just take into account that, since you won't be using hairstyling products, most hairstyles won't hold as well or look the same way as they'd do if you used hairstyling agents. Also, be aware that you may require specific shampooing sessions at times when your hair has been exposed to dirt (e.g. you went camping).

The main drawback is that going solo has an important risk of messing it up. If you are are going solo, you will need to master the Sebum Coating method since any excess sebum will not be removed with shampoo, and shampoo is the best hair-cleaning agent to remove important excesses of sebum accumulation. Hence, in order to avoid the potentially-chaotic scenario of having an excessive sebum buildup occurring on your hair, you must master the Sebum Coating method and have your curls sebuminised like you mean business. Likewise, your daily hair grooming routine may take longer than what it'd otherwise take using hair products, so you have to weigh the pros and cons of going solo.

31) Can I use natural or organic hair products too?

Absolutely. You can decide to only use natural oils and butters on your hair, and you can buy your hair products organic if you so prefer. You can also use natural oils and butters while at times using organic products and other times using regular products for your shampooing and conditioning. Whatever you do, ensure that you abide by the structure of the hair grooming process and adapt your shampooing frequency and hair grooming schedule accordingly.

32) How can I clean my hair with baking soda and vinegar?

There are 2 common household products that are also useful for cleaning your hair: baking soda and vinegar. These 2 products (used in tandem) act like shampoo and can substitute the shampoo on your shampooing days. Their use, however, is fiddly and requires some experimenting to find out the optimal amounts you'll need as well as their optimal frequency of use. Likewise, the application of these 2 products takes longer than that of shampoo, so you may want to use baking soda and vinegar specifically on some days.

To clean your hair with these 2 kitchen products, first use baking soda. Dilute one tablespoon of the baking soda in one glass of warm water. Then, pour the mix on your hair, aiming to have it poured on your scalp and as per the 6 scalp segments (it will get a bit messy though); once the mix is poured, massage the scalp segments as outlined for the shampooing method. Once you have finished massaging (20-second count per segment), rinse the baking soda thoroughly; failure to rinse it well will result in your hair becoming dry or with white particles. After rinsing the baking soda, pour some vinegar on your scalp and locks (the vinegar being previously diluted), aiming to coat your hair with the vinegar. Once your hair is somewhat soaked in vinegar, then rinse the vinegar with water (from the shower bulb). You may skip the thorough rinsing of the vinegar as the vinegar acts a quasi-conditioner, but the only problem is that your hair may end up giving off a strong vinegar smell; leaving the vinegar on your locks without rising may provide an additional cosmetic benefit to your hair, so experiment with both approaches (i.e. rinsing and not rinsing the vinegar) and gauge the results.

The vinegar must be diluted in a container of warm water, and the optimal amounts to be used for your hair will vary. However, a starting point is to dilute half a cup of vinegar into a litre (or 2 pints) of warm water. Then, you can adjust the dilution gradually as you see it benefits your hair. Furthermore, there's no need to finish the whole 1-litre blend of vinegar and water in one session; you may find that only using half of it works optimally. You can use either white vinegar or apple-cider vinegar, and I recommend you to put each blend (baking soda/water and vinegar/water) in containers that have a lid (e.g. empty shampoo bottles) so that you can pour the blends efficiently.

Pros and cons of using this baking soda/vinegar method as opposed to using shampoo for your hair-cleaning stage?

Pros:

- Works just as good as shampoo under normal conditions (i.e. no heavy excesses of sebum buildup).

- The vinegar surprisingly leaves your hair feeling smooth.

- It is as natural as it gets.

Cons:

- Takes much longer to perform than shampooing alone.

- You still need to do the Sebum Coating method on your non-shampooing days (treat the baking soda/vinegar day as a shampooing day).

- If not rinsed thoroughly, the baking soda may dry your hair or leave white particles behind, and the vinegar may leave your hair smelly (of vinegar).

- Will require adjusting your previously-determined hair grooming schedule.

- If you're traveling or not at home, this method is difficult to implement.

- Not strong enough to remove accidents with hairstyling agents (e.g. you mistakenly put too much oil on your hair). For bad cases of excessive residue from hairstyling agents or heavy sebum buildup, use shampoo.

This baking soda/vinegar method is to be regarded as a hair-cleaning method and thus as a secondary action to be implemented for your cleaning stage, and it should be considered a shampooing day every time you proceed with this method. However, if you alternate this method with shampooing days (i.e. days where you actually shampoo and use the baking soda/vinegar method on non-shampooing days), then you can skip the conditioning stage and move on to the styling stage any time you perform the baking soda/vinegar method.

All in all, using the baking soda/vinegar method inserts another variable into your hair grooming that will make your hair grooming routine and schedule more complex. I personally recommend you to stick with the hair grooming method as per Chapter 3 (i.e. shampoo on shampooing days, Sebum Coating method on non-shampooing days), and then, if you are curious, start playing around with the baking soda/vinegar method, inserting a day of its use here and there.

Whatever you do, always have a structure and follow the hair grooming process, otherwise you will get lost in the minutiae and end up not achieving your goal of an awesome mane.

33) What are water-soluble hair products and should I use them?

Water-soluble products are products that are supposedly easier to wash off the hair with the Sebum Coating method (i.e. with water and mechanical friction); they are mostly seen with conditioners (both normal and leave-in) as well as quite a few hairstyling agents (most notably pomade and gel). The problem is that, by becoming water soluble, these products tend to have their functionality altered and the hairstyling results they yield tend to be different to those of their conventional counterparts.

Water-based products are most useful if you're going to completely avoid shampoo and will only rely on the Sebum Coating method (or the baking soda/vinegar method) for your long-term hair cleaning. The thing is, with your hair grooming routine, you will be self-regulating your hair's cleaning regardless of the hair products you use. For example, if you start using a water-soluble pomade, you will very likely find that your shampooing frequency will be reduced somewhat (i.e. you'll shampoo less frequently) if, prior to the water-soluble pomade, you used to use a conventional pomade. The tradeoff is that water soluble pomades do not adequately provide the "greased" look of conventional pomades, so you will be trading the functionality of regular pomade for a lower shampooing frequency.

What's even equally important to know with water-soluble products is that obtaining good results from them is like playing a roulette. You may find a water-soluble product of more benefit while the dude next to you will abhor that product and will need the conventional form of that product. Likewise, remember that your scalp continues to secrete sebum, so you may find that moving to water-soluble agents doesn't necessarily yield any decrease in shampooing frequency as sebum is what's more important to pay attention to for your hair-grooming efforts.

All of the above is why I tell you to trial different hairstyling agents if you're not happy with your current one and to not to focus on the minutiae that complicates matters even more and is subject to further randomness. Start with a hairstyling product that you like (e.g. one you've used in the past) and grab a shampoo and conditioner as per Question 7. Furthermore, smart application of hairstyling agents and conditioners, which is what you've learnt, is much more important than whether a product is water-soluble or not.

Water-soluble hair products will be advertised as such or as "water based". The water-soluble hair product will have ingredients that are indeed water-soluble and that allow the product to be advertised as such.

34) What's the most random awesome-mane personal story that you have?

When I was living in Dubai (United Arab Emirates), I decided to organise a bodyboarding trip to the seacoast in Oman. Oman is one of the neighbouring countries of the United Arab Emirates, and it has a great coastline in the Arabian Sea with some wicked waves (in bodyboarding, you ride waves lying flat on a board).

I was going with a male friend, and we took my car for what was an approximate 1000-mile drive across part of the Arabian Desert. We decided to stop at a random village for a sleepover as it was getting late and driving at night in Oman is crazy as it is, although the skyline as you drive through the Arabian Desert is absolutely stunning. Once we had checked into the only hotel in the village, my buddy and I decided to visit a nearby shisha bar (Arab smoking bar) that was full of locals in their kandoras (a type of full-body vest) and their keffiyehs (a type of head scarf). As soon as we stepped inside the shisha bar, all the locals turned their heads to look at us.

We shrugged off the attention of the local patrons and went about our business getting a hooka (a smoking device) and some of the funky-smelling tobacco that is smoked with the hooka. I don't smoke, but once in a while hitting a shisha bar is fun, and, despite you don't get high from the stuff, it is a pleasurable experience as you sink into the comfortable seats and chat away with your friends while smoking.

The locals kept staring at us, and one of the things that I have learnt when visiting a new country is to always be extra polite and friendly to the locals if you want them to be on your side. However, the whole staring at us was getting well out of order, and, soon enough, the patrons started to move next to us, forming a circle. Mind you, they actually grabbed their seats and moved themselves close to us without saying a single word and staring at us during the whole process. I looked back at them to know what was going on and found out that all of them were, in fact, looking at me and not at my friend.

Homosexuality is banned in Oman, so I knew for sure that we hadn't ended up in a gay bar. The situation was quite worrying because we hardly knew where we were on the map as I had kept driving through a never-ending road that claimed to take us to the Omani seacoast. If something were to happen to us in that shisha bar, nobody would know. The situation was very tense, and I could see through the corner of my eyes how, by now, my buddy stood petrified, and I could swear he had stopped blinking too. We were literally standing in total silence amidst a crowd of about 30 locals who didn't show any facial signs of affection towards us. Moreover, some westerners had been kidnapped recently in Yemen (country next to Oman), so, needless to say, we weren't in the happiest of situations.

Then, I heard a deep masculine voice coming from the back of the bar, asking my friend and I something in Arabic that I didn't understand and that sounded aggressive. Since I hardly spoke Arabic, I then asked politely in English, with my voice trembling but trying to look confident, if he could kindly please repeat what he had said (I emphasised "kindly" and "please" so as to not disturb the angry-sounding local who could potentially kill us and bury our bodies right there). Many westerners have given a bad image of themselves to Omanis, so most locals refuse to speak in English with foreigners and will continue talking in Arabic if they don't like you. I was convinced by now that these guys didn't want to be friends with us.

The aforementioned aggressive-sounding man, somewhere in the invisible back of the bar, then asked me again in Arabic if I spoke Arabic, which I managed to understand, to which I replied (this time in Arabic) that I was sorry but that I didn't speak much of the language. He was addressing me from behind the surrounding crowd, and I could not see him, which added further drama to the situation. He then stepped forward, made his way through the men seating around us and stood in front of me as I remained seated on what, minutes before, was a very comfortable couch.

As soon as he was in front of me, I was able to see how this guy had the bushiest and manliest beard that I had ever seen on anyone, looked about 50 years old and emanated testosterone from every single pore of his skin. Think a darker version of Chuck Norris on a bad day and speaking Arabic.

"I see, my friend", he said, surprising all of us in the room as he had decided to speak those words in English.

He paused for a few seconds, the room in total silence. These seconds seemed like an eternity to me, and I just stood there frozen like a bag of broccoli left overnight in the freezer. I was waiting for the bad news despite he had called me his friend.

"You have nice hair, my friend", he then said, breaking the agonising silence that filled the room.

I could not believe it; I was shocked and convinced that he was just giving me a nice compliment to sugarcoat my impending death. He then looked back to the crowd, said something in Arabic, and all the other men started smiling and shouting stuff in joy. The Chuck Norris look-alike then grabbed a chair and sat a mere inches away from me, sporting the biggest and friendliest of smiles.

"What nation you are, my friend?" he asked in broken English.

Still in shock, I managed to say my country of origin. He continued to smile and asked my name; I told him my name, and he then tried to pronounce it, not sounding at all like I had said it (mind you, my name is hard to pronounce as it is). The crowd laughed, and he encouraged me to teach him to pronounce the "-ge" in Rogelio. He got it right on the third attempt.

"You have nice hair, my friend Rogelio."

"Shookran ekteer", I said in Arabic so as to thank him for his kind words.

He smiled as so did the men in the crowd.

He then ordered the guy who was acting as the de facto waiter to bring us more funky tobacco to put on our hookah as well as some huge plates of food for my friend and I to feast on. My new local buddy was literally 2 inches away from me, talking constantly in his broken English while my friend (the one who came with me for the trip) ignored the 2 of us and munched away the food we were brought.

My new buddy was talking about how his sons had hair just like mine and how he would crop their hair to a #2 with a hair clipper that he had. He told me in an amusing manner how his daughters had very curly hair like his and that the girls were always complaining about their hair. While the local traditions frown upon talking about one's wife to another man (especially to a foreigner), he told me that his wife had beautiful straight hair and that he had hoped his daughters would have inherited their mother's hair and not his.

We spent the next 4 hours chatting about hair, hair-related stuff, soccer, local traditions, western culture and joked about our cultural differences. The image that the media in the West gives about Arab people is completely distorted; they made my friend and I feel at home, which is pretty much the same vibe that I have encountered during my life in the Middle East.

We finished off our ramblings and the food devouring, and we went back to our hotel to get some sleep. The next day, we found out that someone had filled up the fuel tank of my car and had cleaned the car's chassis from the desert dust accumulated overnight, all without me knowing anything about it. We also had a box full of water bottles and food waiting for us in the reception of the hotel. As it goes, my new local friend had left a note in reception thanking me for the conversation we had the previous night and for the hair tips and advice I gave him for his children. He had ordered the taking care of my car, the buying for us of provisions for our trip, and he had even sorted out and paid for accommodation for my friend and I to stay in a 4-star hotel in the seaside village we were heading to for our bodyboarding trip! It turned out that he was one of the most respected tribal members in the region, and he had made a few phone calls to make our trip better. Call that luck!

Even though this personal story is one of those rare occurrences, I have had other less exotic yet similar stories happening with greater frequency. It is human nature, regardless of culture or beliefs, to show an interest and appreciation for anything that is unique, different (in an admirable way) and inspiring. While these 3 traits are worthy of admiration and emulation in today's society, average Joes and Johns fail to paradoxically show interest in pursuing them because they don't have the optimal tools and knowledge to do so. Pursuing your awesome mane is one of those small things in life that is based on having the optimal tools and knowledge, and its accomplishment will have you adding another success to an overall better life full of achievements, uniqueness and admiration, as it has for me.

35) Are there more things I should know outside of those in this book to get my awesome mane?

No, not to get your awesome mane. I have written this book with an emphasis on the male who wants a great-looking mane with convenience. You only need to look at the 9-Minute Perfect Mane routine to see the emphasised blend of great results with convenience: you have learnt all the details that go with the actions needed to implement the 9-Minute Perfect Mane routine, and you can easily implement all the actions in 9 minutes or less. I have designed this routine so that you invest 9 minutes of your time to be able to leave your house with an awesome mane. I could have instead designed a Perfect Mane routine that was attained in 60 minutes, but then, how convenient and relevant would it have been to a modern 21st century curly haired male like you and I? What's more is that I have experimented with 60-minute grooming routines and found no real extra benefit from what I could otherwise achieve with a 9-minute routine.

I am a strong believer in the Pareto principle. Applied in a non-economic sense, this principle proposes that 80% of results can be achieved with 20% of the 100% of efforts needed to obtain 100% of results. In this book, I bring you exactly this, only that, with this 20% of efforts, you will actually be getting about 95% of results; and that's with 100% of the results being super-duper fabulous diva curls, so you are a mere 5% short of getting your Sex in the City "oh dear, I can't believe it's so awesomely curly" curls. Or in others words, you are getting your awesome mane (95%), and the remaining 5% is not worth the effort unless you want to remove convenience from your daily hair-management equation.

Following on from the above, however, I'd like to briefly cover the other things that you can do to tap into the remaining 5% of the aforementioned 100% results.

Deep condition frequently

Curly hair is very hard to over-moisturise especially if you fall into curl types Type III and above. Deep conditioning is a form of sealing in extra moisture into the hair and is of special benefit to damaged hair. Damaged hair occurs from subpar hair care as well as from straightening, relaxing or dying your curls, which is not something you will be doing anyway with your awesome mane.

Because deep conditioning is literally a heavy-duty form of conditioning, it requires more application time and effort than a normal conditioner does. I have experimented with deep conditioners and haven't experienced any major benefits from doing them at any rate or frequency because my hair has already been taken care of with optimal hair grooming and caring as detailed in this book. If you abide by the concept of an awesome mane, you seldom need deep conditioners (if at all).

However, if your current hair has been cared badly or has been straightened, relaxed or dyed, then using a deep conditioner to jump-start your awesome mane is advised if you want to keep your current hair, although, for best physical hair results, I recommend you to instead start your awesome mane journey with a fresh and virgin batch of hair (i.e. cut your damaged hair).

If you want to use a deep conditioner even though you already have an awesome mane, you can deep condition anywhere from once a week to once a month, and try to do it on your shampooing day, swapping your normal conditioner for the deep conditioner.

Go into more detail about profiling your hair

I could tell you to also classify your hair according to your strand thickness, protein sensitivity, strand porosity or really dig into the coil factor. At the end of the day, however, you'd be even more confused than when you started reading and would be feeling like you are reading a manual for girls.

All the important stuff that you need to know so as to profile your hair is in this book, and I have written it so that it is especially relevant to the lifestyle-conscious modern male who wants great convenient curly hair (i.e. you). I have written this book as a modern male for the modern male, and it is my belief that you only need to go as far as the tested basics in hair profiling to further define your hair management and achieve your awesome mane.

Split hairs about what goes on when you sleep

I could easily tell you to wear a silk scarf around your head when you go to bed, or I could tell you to avoid sleeping on the sides of your head so as to not offset the uber-curvylicious definition of your curls. By the same token, I could also tell you to sleep vertically and not on a bed because, apparently, this enhances the delta waves produced in the subaquatic region of the phospholipid membrane in the left hemisphere of your brain, and this has been proven to increase concentration levels by 1.1% in sleep-deprived iguanas. At the end of the day, though, you'd have to weigh the pros and cons of what you do.

Sure, when you have your head rubbing against a pillow for 6 to 9 hours, your hair will take some beating. However, I will tell you that impairing your sleep with trivial stuff (e.g. scarves to elaborately protect the hair) will affect your health (including hair) more than any small benefit that obsessing about your mane when you go to bed will yield. Sleep is essential to health and a great life, and optimal sleep should be very high up in your list of priorities, higher than hair actually.

I have done the whole pre-bed routine of covering my mane with weird stuff, soaking my hair in gooish products and more. The result was an uncomfortable night and bad sleep, just to have my curls look a little bit better than if I had gone to bed as I have outlined in this book. You tell me, how am I going to incorporate my awesome mane into a better life if I am failing to optimise adequate rest and sleep, the latter being one of the foundations to a great life?

As I have suggested in the chapter "Hair Care: Looking After Your Healthy Awesome Mane", tie your hair at night into a ponytail or bun if your hair is long enough. If your hair isn't long enough to tie it, you can wear a sleeping cap or do-rag on your head to help minimise the friction on your mane from rubbing your head on the pillow during sleep. If you decide to wear a sleeping cap or do-rag, make sure that it is secured properly and that it doesn't interfere with your sleeping comfort, and you can also coat your curls with some conditioner prior to putting on the sleeping cap or do-rag. Lastly, buy yourself a satin or silk pillow case to minimise head friction, and call it a day. Enjoy your sleep and, when you get up, do the 9-Minute Perfect Mane routine; voila, you have your awesome mane ready to take the day. Tried, tested and guaranteed.

My personal experience

My awesome mane journey was full of questions. I even thought of giving up at different points as, after all, I was alone in my endeavours; I was trying to achieve something that was, at the time, seen as impossible by most curly men: aesthetic curly hair that one would be satisfied and proud to have. Despite experiencing some negative episodes in the beginning, I was determined to continue with my journey as I would reach, time and time again, to the same strong-minded and determined attitude that I had decided to develop when I started addressing that which was mine and which would help me to become a better man. Had it not been for the attitude I had developed, I would have never made it through and achieved my awesome mane; hence the reason for dedicating a whole chapter to the mental part of achieving great-looking curly hair.

I like to use inspiring people as references whenever I am trying to accomplish a goal that I have set myself. I dislike idolising or having heroes; rather, I like to surround myself with people whom I can learn from and be inspired by. I am talking about hard-working, determined people: mere individuals who have decided to pursue a lifelong path to bring benefit to themselves and to others. In my eyes, those are the real life "heroes" and "idols", yet, somehow, being a hard-working, determined, noble, creative, humble, fair, strong, wise, dedicated and passionate man has lost its relevance and importance in today's society.

I have had and continue to have many references and sources of inspiration. They are not popular in the strictest of terms. They do not appear in magazines or TV ads. They do not have legions of groupies chasing them, and they certainly don't earn millions influencing others in their life decisions. They are average men and women whom I have met during my travels and life experiences; individuals who have inspired me in one way or another, allowing me to adapt what I learnt from them to my own particular case and life. In fact, I have been able to gather more life inspiration and lessons from a 60-year-old man who owns a seaside kiosk in my hometown and who wakes up at 5:00 AM every Sunday to open his business than I have ever gathered from The Situation or Soulja Boy, yet the latter 2 are huge social influencers (kudos to them for being so, though).

In the past and even to this day, all I have had to do when I was feeling down was to look at those real-life men and women whom I have met during my lifetime and who have achieved great things in their lives despite their paths to success being plagued with questions, obstacles, mob mentality, and having to test and then test some more to achieve results. It is these people that have ultimately helped me to visualise the path to a life of continuous self-actualization and whose lessons have served me as deterrents to any questions or pessimistic thoughts that I've encountered during my awesome mane journey and during the whole journey that life is.

The questions in this chapter are the ones that I have encountered or that others who came to me for answers have encountered. Most importantly, do remember at all times that this book is your tool to your awesome mane and that all the knowledge you need is inside this book. No amount of questions should deviate you from your journey, and you will achieve your awesome mane goal if you put your mind to it!

9) Wrapping It All Up: You Are Now Ready, My Friend

"Love is a better teacher than a sense of duty"

Albert Einstein

That is it. If you are reading these lines, you have finished the book, and you are now ready to start your awesome mane journey. Of course, go back to this book as often as you need as you continue your journey, and do keep in mind that obtaining a great head of curly hair has an important component of trial and error: you will have to find out some elements of your awesome mane via testing and observation (e.g. shampooing frequency) as these elements are unique to you, the same way that your self-puzzle is also unique to you.

Your awesome mane has a physical part and a mental part. Chapters 2 to 5 specifically address the physical part, and Chapter 6 specifically addresses the mental part. Overall though, both parts to an awesome mane are constantly referenced in all chapters because having the right mindset will be key in developing the physical part of your awesome mane and obtaining physical results will be key in reinforcing the mindset that you will need to achieve an awesome mane. One (physical part) cannot go without the other (mental part).

Whether you have hated your curly hair in the past, succumbed to buzz cuts due to lack of knowledge, never been inspired, or never had your curls as you wanted them to look like, this book provides you with answers so as to provide you with an overall solution: to finally be satisfied with your curly hair (i.e. have your awesome mane). I have been where you are right now, and I would not have written a book about all of this if I didn't know that it can certainly be achieved by a modern male and that the benefits of having an awesome mane are just too great to be neglecting the stuff that comes to you naturally.

Take your time, and see your journey as a path full of steps to be achieved and actions to be implemented. Achieving any goal you set yourself requires the right tools and the right knowledge, correct, but it too requires a planned journey, a way of doing, a series of intelligent actions; and an awesome mane is no less. Start your journey by first knowing your curly hair (Chapter 2), then proceed with sorting out its day-to-day management (hair grooming, Chapter 3), then think long term (hair care, Chapter 4), then put the icing on the cake (Chapter 5). In the process, build and reinforce your attitude, search for inspiration, and solidify your motivation (Chapter 6). Any questions or unsure about anything? Chapters 7 and 8 will then fill in the blanks.

To further ensure that you know what to look out for and learn in each of the chapters of this book, I will now, below these lines, go through the most important stuff that needs to be extracted from each of the chapters.

What you should be picking up from each chapter

Chapter 1 – Introduction: The Start Of An Awesome Mane Journey

Understand what the Awesome Mane concept is, what it entails and spans, and what are its rules. Know that an awesome mane has 2 parts: a physical part and a mental part. Likewise, know that you, as a male, are made up of personal traits (i.e. pieces) that altogether make your self-puzzle (i.e. who you are). Your awesome mane is about addressing a piece of your self-puzzle, which is why it requires a certain mental part. You are not just improving the looks of your hair; you are improving yourself as a modern male.

Ultimately, know why you want to do this. If you are at a time in your life that you cannot begin your awesome mane journey straightaway, then delay its start. Do not give this a half-baked effort; start your journey only when you are ready.

Chapter 2 – Curly Hair 101: Know Your Waves, Coils Or Kinks

Understand what curly hair is and that it is expressed in 5 types, and then identify your curl type. Understand what the extended and visible lengths are and work them out, being aware that ultimately it is your extended length category that is most relevant to your hair grooming efforts, so do identify which category your extended hair length falls into.

While your curl type, 2 hair lengths and extended hair length category are the most important elements to know when it comes to 101-type knowledge of your hair, there are some smaller, much-less-relevant tidbits that are good to have in the back of your mind as they will help you to fully grasp the content of the rest of the chapters.

Chapter 3 – Hair Grooming: Get Those Curls Looking Great

It is very important for you to know what the hair grooming process entails, to know each of the 3 stages in depth and to know and be acquainted with the secondary actions. Your hair grooming routine, portrayed as the 9-Minute Perfect Mane routine, is comprised of 3 stages implemented in a sequential and synchronised manner, and your hair grooming routine is to be done every day albeit modifying the secondary actions to be performed in each stage.

Your hair grooming routine always follows the same stages: cleaning, conditioning and styling. In the first stage, cleaning, there are 2 secondary actions that are alternated according to the day: shampooing and the Sebum Coating method. In the second stage, conditioning, you have 3 secondary actions: use a normal conditioner, skip the normal conditioner, or take advantage of the hair-conditioning synergy yielded by the Sebum Coating method as used to clean the hair. Lastly, for the third stage, styling, you have a range of hairstyles and hairstyling agents available, and you must also understand how to implement your styling, from drying your hair to how to apply your chosen hairstyling agents.

You should regard the Sebum Coating method as the extremely valuable secondary action that it is. The Sebum Coating method essentially acts as a shampoo and as a normal conditioner, and it is used on the days that no shampoo is used. Because it simultaneously cleans and conditions the hair, the Sebum Coating method not only substitutes for a shampoo but also substitutes for a normal conditioner, hence the stages of cleaning and conditioning can be merged on non-shampooing days.

It is your shampooing frequency that determines each of the stages' secondary actions to be implemented on both your shampooing and non-shampooing days, and it is the shampooing frequency that you should be building your hair grooming routine and schedule from. Thus, before building your routine, you must find out your shampooing frequency, and in the meantime use a generic hair grooming routine as recommended and per the table on Appendix XXII: use a shampoo, normal conditioner and any hairstyling agents on your shampooing days, and use the Sebum Coating method, a leave-in conditioner and any hairstyling agents on your non-shampooing days. On the days that you shampoo, practise the 9-Minute Perfect Mane routine so that you start becoming efficient in your hair grooming actions.

Once you have found out your shampooing frequency, it is then that you can start modifying your hair grooming actions from the generic routine that you had been using up until then. In terms of hair products, you should be buying initially a shampoo with a sulfate-type ingredient, a normal conditioner, a leave-in conditioner, a hairstyling agent of your choice and a wide-tooth comb. Once you have a solid hair grooming routine, you can start buying more hair products and different brands if you so wish to. You can also purchase a hair dryer but bear in mind that this hairstyling tool is to be used occasionally and not daily.

Chapter 4 – Hair Care: Looking After Your Healthy Awesome Mane

Hair care should be seen as a strategy to use to ensure your awesome mane for the long term. The health of your awesome mane (defined as its good looks and undamaged state) is maintained by using proactive and reactive measures as well as by your optimal intake of nutrients.

With your awesome mane, you will be facing 3 main issues on a daily basis: dry hair, tangled hair and hair loss, and each of these issues has its set of proactive and reactive measures to be neutralised with. Thus, not only do you need to know your awesome mane issues but also your hair care measures, and you should be selecting those measures that are appropriate for your personal case, making sure to abide by their frequent use as part of your overall hair care strategy.

I have also given you the nutritional approach that I use for my awesome mane. It is important that you are aware that having an optimised diet and supplementation regimen aids in maximising your awesome mane potential, thus you can take the advice in my nutritional approach to design your own diet and supplementation regimen, always consulting first with your doctor before modifying your diet or deciding to take any nutritional supplements. Your health comes first, and having optimal health is essential to achieving the greatest-looking awesome mane that you can possibly own.

Chapter 5 – Achieving The Physical Part: Putting Your Mane Together

Hair grooming and hair care are the essential aspects of the physical part of your awesome mane; anything that you do outside of these 2 physical aspects will be the icing on the cake. Thus, this fifth chapter deals with everything that encompasses putting a form and shape to your awesome mane.

As a curly dude, you have many hairstyles to choose from, but it is imperative that you are realistic and can tell what is personally doable as a hairstyle and what isn't. Not only do you have 3 hairstyles recommended for your specific curl type but also the hairstyles recommended for the curl types nearing yours can suit you very well, so you certainly have hairstyles to choose from.

Now that you have an awesome mane, you should not be settling for anyone cutting your hair. Whenever you want to go for a haircut, go through the points given to you in this chapter. If you find a hairdresser or barber whom you are happy with, then build a relationship with him/her so as to get the most efficient hairdressing service that you can find.

In terms of hair accessories, feel free to use any of the ones mentioned, but always remember that hair accessories should be there to enhance your awesome mane, not to detract from it.

The last section of this chapter gives you the recommended steps and actions to start and pave your awesome mane journey with. You can deviate from the recommended flow if you want to, but the flow I have given you is the one tried and tested.

Chapter 6 – The Mental Part: Attitude, Lifestyle And Making It Awesome

After reading all the chapters dedicated to the physical part of an awesome, a chapter about the mental part is in due order. Throughout the previous chapters, you have already read about the attitude and other mental aspects of an awesome mane, so it is in this chapter where you learn in depth all about the mental part of an awesome mane. Not only do you learn per se but this chapter will also serve to ingrain the mental fortitude and attitude necessary to successfully keep your awesome mane for the rest of your life.

Apart from the above, there's a self-actualising side to an awesome mane: you can regard the achievement of your awesome mane as part of instilling in yourself a success-seeking and self-improving mentality. You can continue to milk the positivity created by having achieved this goal you set yourself (i.e. an awesome mane) and thus put yourself on a life path that encourages achieving goals and being successful. The positivity stemming from achieving an awesome mane is a superb benefit by itself, and I have seen and experienced how doing what you are about to do can bring much satisfaction and value to one's life. Ergo, at the very least

I'd like for you to be aware of this extra benefit that you can go on to realise and develop once your awesome mane goal has been achieved.

Lastly, and in a more entertaining manner, an awesome mane is sexy, and you will get extra attention wherever you go, so I'd rather prepare you for what is to come once you get a head of luscious curls!

Chapter 7 – Hair Mythology: Don't Be Fooled Any More

Well, this chapter is all about debunking myths. You will possibly be guilty of some of these myths as so was I when I started my awesome mane journey many years ago. Consequently, it is extremely valuable for you to be able to tell true from false as time efficiency is of the utmost value in your awesome mane journey. I have wasted much time with myths and nonsense prior to starting and in the beginning of my awesome mane journey, so I don't want you to go through the same inefficient ordeal. Simply keep all these myths in the back of your mind during your journey.

Chapter 8 – Questions & Answers: Because They Will Come

Questions will come; I know that because I too had questions when I started. Most questions that crop up during your journey will only need a quick browsing through the chapter related to the newly-cropped-up question to be solved.

The questions that you can read in this chapter are those miscellaneous ones that I have asked myself or that those whom I have advised have asked me at one time or another. However, the worst question that you can ask yourself is the one that leads to mental defeat, so I have ensured to provide you with my personal experience and how I have used real-life inspiration to stay put and determined to achieve my goals. If I can do it after having lived in different countries and having a modern lifestyle, and if my 60-year-old friend can wake up every Sunday at 5:00 AM to open his seaside kiosk, then rest assured that you too can achieve your goal of an awesome mane.

Chapter 9 – Wrapping It All Up: You Are Now Ready, My Friend & Appendix

This current chapter that you are reading has The Curly Hair Book: Or How Men Can Now Rock Their Waves, Coils And Kinks coming to fruition. Each chapter is summarised so that you can know what to specifically pick up and learn during your reading.

Below these lines, you will find the last section of this chapter and of all chapters, and it is where I will give you my last words. Then, the Appendix will be all that there is left for you to read in this book; the Appendix contains all the illustrative material used throughout the book, including tables, photographs and drawings. Thus, the Appendix is the part of this book where you can find all used material that can be glanced at any time for a quick view.

Last words from yours truly

Without your involvement, this book would be just that, a book. I have written this book for you and for the rest of men who have waves, coils and kinks for hair. A population segment for which each single male has had to battle with his hair from birth; you and I know very well what it is like to have curly hair, and we can certainly relate to what other fellow curly haired males can be going through too. Thus, this special follicular commonality unites us together just like all social groups are tailored around central attributes that bring people together: favourite sport teams, literary tastes, political beliefs or music affiliations. In retrospect, we own an attribute that we can all talk to each other about, being able to relate to one another and help each other to become better.

Be part of spreading the word. Tell and share with other curly men what an awesome mane is, let them know that there is more to life than buzz cuts and dead rats. Enlighten those who are not privileged as of yet to have read what you have read, and show them the optimal "curly male" way with this book and with what you have leant and acquired.

Through the years, I have seen how a curly male's self-confidence vastly improves upon fixing his curly hair; an asset in itself that is far too commonly deemed as a liability and not the other way around. Furthermore, rejecting and hating that which comes to one naturally is an awful way to live one's life, and achieving an awesome mane is a fantastic way to turn the tables and improve oneself. This is why I have been aiming to spread the word now for quite some time, and it is why I decided to take a step further in my peculiar goal and write this book. Without you, your involvement and the rest of curly men who are yet to be shown the way, this book would not have a point to make, a reason for being, a purpose behind. Together, we can spread the word and strengthen our lives and the lives of others; never forget that life has a beautiful way of rewarding those who help others.

By all means, this book is part of my overall goal of spreading the word, and there's more to this coming, which is why I encourage your involvement too. Of course, you can find me online at my site, on Facebook, on Twitter and more that is to come soon. For now, these are the places where I hang out:

www.manlycurls.com

www.facebook.com/ManlyCurls

https://twitter.com/ManlyCurls

I appreciate your input, comments, reviews, feedback and anything that you'd like to say and/or think that can be done. More so, I very much welcome your progress updates and for the time being our hanging-out place is my site Manly Curls, though do stay tuned for more. I currently have a section where I feature some of our readers, and you are welcome to be featured in this section too.

This is my first time writing an actual book, and I'm certainly popping my book-author cherry by publishing this book. It's quite the thrill and responsibility, and all I can say is that it has been an utter joy and satisfaction to have written this book. I have truly enjoyed this experience, and I have written this book in the wildest of places (4 countries) and in the most confined of situations (e.g. hand writing for 4 hours straight in a plane because my laptop battery died while a child in the next seat was crying nonstop). Really, it has been some wild and awesome time.

I am specifically writing this last section after having written all of the book; I purposely left this paragraph till last, and these are now my last words. Not only has this being an immensely-satisfying literary journey but I am also proud of this book, and I am 100% convinced that it will be of value to you because this has been my precise motive from the very start. Moreover, it is an absolute pleasure and privilege to share this book with you and have you reading it, and, while I've already thanked you in the beginning of the book, I'd like to thank you again for having taken the time to read my words and believe in my message. I am the first one who believes in you and who knows that you will indeed achieve your goal of an awesome mane and any other goal that you set yourself in life, for you are one of us now.

Take action, stay determined, and strive to be an overall better man, fellow awesome mane friend.

All the best.

Rogelio

Appendix

AWESOME MANE	
Physical	*Mental*
Hair grooming	Attitude
Hair care	Social references
Haircut/Hairstyle	Inspiration
Hair accessories	Motivation
Hair products	Self-puzzle enhancement

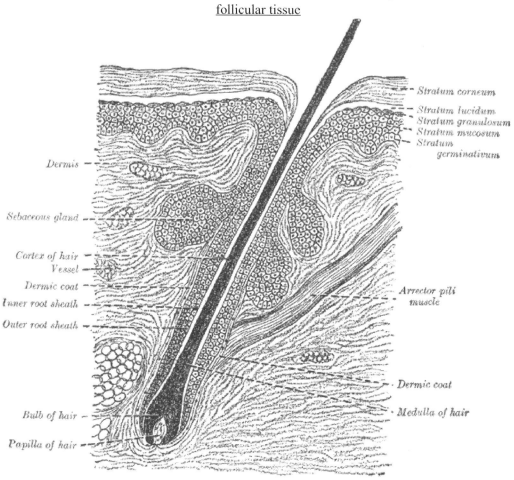

Stratum corneum

Stratum lucidum
Stratum granulosum
Stratum mucosum
Stratum germinativum

Dermis

Sebaceous gland

Cortex of hair
Vessel
Dermic coat
Inner root sheath
Outer root sheath

Arrector pili muscle

Dermic coat

Medulla of hair

Bulb of hair

Papilla of hair

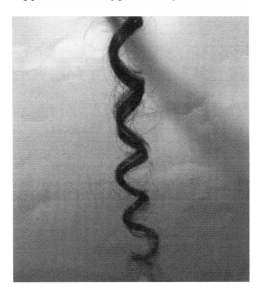

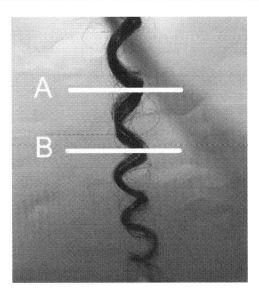

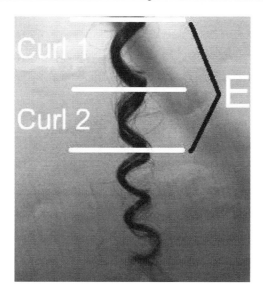

Appendix VI – 4 full curls identified in a curly haired lock

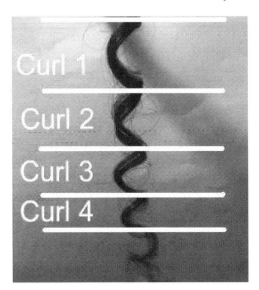

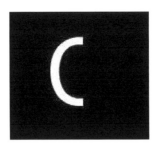

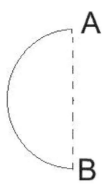

Appendix IX – Example of several typical curly haired locks

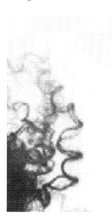

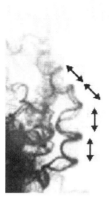

FRONT OF HEAD

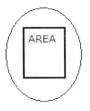

AREA

BACK OF HEAD

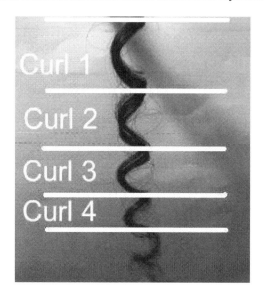

	CURLY HAIR TYPES				
	I	II	III	IV	V
Common name	Wavy	Wavy/Loose Curls	Coiled/Ringlets	Kinky/Kinky Curly	Kinky/Afro
Vertical Length of curl	2 to 3 inches	1 to 2 inches	0.5 to 1 inch	0.25 to 0.5 inches	up to 0.25 inches
Male references	Hugh Grant Antonio Banderas George Clooney	Adrian Grenier Matthew Mcconaughey Nick Jonas	Will Ferrell Justin Timberlake John Turturro	Corbin Bleu Jaden Smith Troy Polamalu	Cuba Gooding Jr. Will Smith Morgan Freeman
Shampooing frequency	Moderate	Moderate	Low	Low	Very low
Need for extra conditioning (normal + leave-in conditioner)	Low	Moderate	Moderate	High	High

	CURLY HAIR TYPES				
	I	II	III	IV	V
Common name	Wavy	Wavy/Loose Curls	Coiled/Ringlets	Kinky/Kinky Curly	Kinky/Afro
Vertical Length of curl	2 to 3 inches	1 to 2 inches	0.5 to 1 inch	0.25 to 0.5 inches	-0.25 inches
Male references	Hugh Grant Antonio Banderas George Clooney	Adrian Grenier Matthew Mcconaughey Nick Jonas	Will Ferrell Justin Timberlake John Turturro	Corbin Bleu Jaden Smith Troy Polamalu	Cuba Gooding Jr. Will Smith Morgan Freeman
Shampooing frequency	Moderate	Moderate	Low	Low	Very low
Need for extra conditioning (normal + leave-in conditioner)	Low	Moderate	Moderate	High	High

224

EXTENDED HAIR LENGTH	
Hair length (inches)	Hair length category
-0.125	Near-shaved
0.125 – 2	Short
2 – 6	Medium
6+	Long

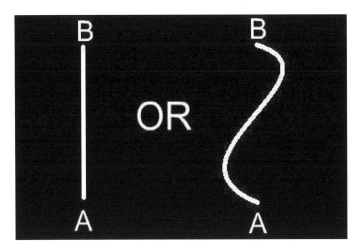

Appendix XVII – Timespans needed to grow each curl type to each visible hair length (months)

	VISIBLE HAIR LENGTH				
	Shaved	2 inches	4 inches	6 inches	12 inches
Straight hair	0	4	8	12	24
Type I	0	5	10	15	30
Type II	0	6	12	18	36
Type III	0	8	16	24	48
Type IV	0	10	20	30	60
Type V	0	12	24	36	72

Appendix XVIII – Estimation of extended hair length at each visible hair length (inches)

	VISIBLE HAIR LENGTH				
	Shaved	2 inches	4 inches	6 inches	12 inches
Straight hair	0	2	4	6	12
Type I	0	2.5	5	7.5	15
Type II	0	3	6	9	18
Type III	0	4	8	12	24
Type IV	0	5	10	15	30
Type V	0	6	12	18	36

STAGES	SECONDARY ACTIONS			
Cleaning	Shampooing	Sebum Coating method		
Conditioning	Use normal conditioner	Sebum Coating method	Skip conditioning	
Styling	Use leave-in conditioner	Use hairstyling agent/s	Put hair into hairstyle	Dry hair

Appendix XX – Typical shampooing frequency per curl type and hair length category (High= 1 on/1 off, Very low= 1 on/7 off)

	CURLY HAIR TYPES				
	Type I	Type II	Type III	Type IV	Type V
Near-shaved	High	High	Moderate	Moderate	Moderate
Short	High	Moderate	Moderate	Low	Low
Medium	Moderate	Moderate	Low	Low	Very low
Long	Moderate	Low	Low	Very low	Very low

Appendix XXI – Example of a weekly schedule according to a 1 on/1 off shampooing frequency

	Monday	Tuesday	Wednesday	Thursday	Friday	Saturday	Sunday
Shampoo	On	Off	On	Off	On	Off	On
Sebum Coating method	Off	On	Off	On	Off	On	Off
Conditioner	On	Off	On	Off	On	Off	On
Leave-in (as styling agent)	Off	On	Off	On	Off	On	Off
Style	Yes	Yes	Yes	Yes	Yes	Yes	Yes
Time Taken (minutes)	8.7 mins	4.5 mins	8.7 mins	4.5 mins	8.7 mins	4.5 mins	8.7 mins

STAGES	SHAMPOOING DAY	NON-SHAMPOOING DAY
Cleaning	Shampoo	Sebum Coating method
Conditioning	Normal conditioner	*(dual action)*
Styling	Yes	Yes
Leave-in conditioner?	No *(style with other hairstyling agent)*	Yes *(style with leave-in + other hairstyling agent)*

SHORT-LENGTH HAIR (UP TO 2 INCHES)	Type I	Type II	Type III	Type IV	Type V
Shampoo	1 on 1 off	1 on 1 off	1 on 2 off	1 on 2 off	1 on 3 off
Conditioner	Every shampooing day	Every shampooing day	Every shampooing day + 50% off days	Every shampooing day + 50% off days	Every shampooing day + 50% off days
Sebum Coating method	Every non-shampooing day	Every non-shampooing day	Every non-shampooing day	Every non-shampooing day	Every non-shampooing day
Leave-in	Every non-shampooing day	Every non-shampooing day	Every non-shampooing day	Every non-shampooing day	Every non-shampooing day
Hairstyling agents	Wax/Pomades/Gel/Mousse	Wax/Pomades/Gel/Mousse	Wax/Pomades/Gel/Mousse/Spray/Pomade	Leave-in/Gel/Oils/Styling creams/Pomade	Leave-in/Oils/Styling cream
Combing	Wide-tooth/Fingers	Wide-tooth/Fingers	Wide-tooth/Fingers	Wide-tooth/Fingers	Wide-tooth/Fingers
Suitable hairstyle	Spikes	Caesar Cut	Faux Hawk	High and Tight	Buzz Cut
Ease of growing to medium length	Easy	Easy	Easy	Moderate	Moderate
Tangling risk	Low	Low	Low	Moderate	Moderate
Ability to puff out	Low	Low	Moderate	High	High
Damp vs. Dry Effect	Barely	Barely	Mild	Mild	Moderate
Drying method	Towel/Palmed Shakeout	Towel/Palmed Shakeout	Towel/Palmed Shakeout	Towel/Palmed Shakeout	Towel/Palmed Shakeout

MEDIUM-LENGTH HAIR (2 TO 6 INCHES)

	Type I	Type II	Type III	Type IV	Type V
Shampoo	1 on 2 off	1 on 2 off	1 on 3 off	1 on 4 off	1 on 4 off
Conditioner	Every shampooing day	Every shampooing day	Every shampooing day + 50% off days	Every shampooing day + 50% off days	Every shampooing day + 75% off days
Sebum Coating method	Every non-shampooing day	Every non-shampooing day	Every non-shampooing day	Every non-shampooing day	Every non-shampooing day
Leave-in	Every non-shampooing day	Every non-shampooing day	Every non-shampooing day	Daily	Daily
Hairstyling agents	Wax/Pomades/Gel/Mousse	Pomades/Gel/Spray/Mousse/Leave-in made	Leave-cream/Mousse/Pomade	Leave-in/Gels/Oils/Styling cream/Pomade	Leave-in/Oils/Styling cream
Combing	Wide-tooth/Fingers	Wide-tooth/Fingers	Wide-tooth/Fingers	Wide-tooth/Fingers	Wide-tooth/Fingers
Suitable hairstyle	Side Fringe	Side Swept	Jewfro	Shake & Go	Afro
Ease of growing to long length	Easy	Moderate	Moderate	Hard	Hard
Tangling risk	Low	Low	Moderate	High	High
Ability to puff out	Low	Low	Moderate	High	High
Damp vs. Dry Effect	Barely	Mild	Mild	Moderate	Intense
Drying method	Towel/Shakeout	Towel/Shakeout	Towel/Shakeout	Towel/Shakeout	Towel/Shakeout

LONG-LENGTH HAIR (OVER 6 INCHES)	Type I	Type II	Type III	Type IV	Type V
Shampoo	1 on 2 off	1 on 3 off	1 on 4 off	1 on 5 off	1 on 6 off
Conditioner	Every shampooing day	Every shampooing day + 50% off days	Every shampooing day + 50% off days	Every shampooing day + 75% off days	Every shampooing day + 75% off days
Sebum Coating method	Every non-shampooing day	Every non-shampooing day	Every non-shampooing day	Every non-shampooing day	Every non-shampooing day
Leave-in	Daily	Daily	Daily	Daily	Daily
Hairstyling agents	Pomades/Gel/Mousse/Leave-in/Spray	Pomades/Gel/Mousse/Leave-in/Spray	Pomades/Gel/Mousse/Pomade/Oils in/Gel/Styling cream	Leave-in/Gels/Oils/Styling cream	Leave-in/Oils/Styling cream
Suitable hairstyle	Shoulder Length	Jim Morrison	Hanging locks	Beyond Shoulder Length	Braids
Combing	Wide-tooth/Fingers	Wide-tooth/Fingers	Wide-tooth/Fingers	Wide-tooth/Fingers	Wide-tooth/Fingers
Ease of growing to very long lengths	Moderate	Moderate	Hard	Hard	Hard
Tangling risk	Moderate	Moderate	High	High	High
Ability to puff out	Low	Low	Moderate	High	High
Damp vs. Dry Effect	Barely	Mild	Mild	Moderate	Intense
Drying method	Towel/Shakeout	Towel/Shakeout	Towel/Shakeout	Towel/Shakeout	Towel/Shakeout

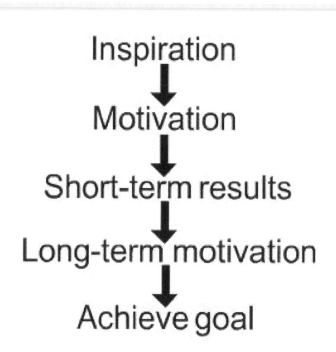

Improve hair ➡ Improve physique ➡ Improve other areas

Made in the USA
San Bernardino, CA
06 February 2015